Dare to Care is a wonderful book: ... compassion. I warmly recommen ... especially those in the early years ... before too much of the "hidden curriculum" has hardened their outlook on the profession.

– **Peter Sullivan, MD**
Emeritus Professor Pediatrics, University of Oxford Medical School, UK
Associate Dean Postgraduate Medicine, University of Oxford Medical School, UK

Dare to Care is a heartwarming book that uses letters from Dr. Bonhoeffer to his goddaughter, a resident physician. Through these letters, Dr. Bonhoeffer imparts his wisdom, experience and, most important, his compassion not only to his goddaughter but to each of us. Whether you're a medical student or seasoned physician, this book will remind you of why you became a physician.

– **James Doty, MD**
Professor of Neurosurgery, Stanford University School of Medicine
Founder and Director, The Center for Compassion and Altruism Research and Education (CCARE)

A great book! It gives us – medics and patients – a simple truth that everyone knows, but almost nobody bothers about in actual practice: Healing is not only about scientific facts and medical technology (which are important enough); it is also about love. This book contains more wisdom than a bookshelf of recent publications in philosophy.

– **Olaf Müller, PhD**
Professor of Philosophy of Science and Nature, Humboldt University, Berlin, Germany

This book is so much deeper than just a dialogue between a physician and a medical student; it cuts right to both the essence of healing and what it means to be human.

– **Thom Hartmann**

Nationally syndicated American radio personality, New York Times best-selling author, former psychotherapist

In *Dare to Care*, the authors astutely describe the exquisite art of medicine. Physician burnout and disillusionment are often the result of extreme focus on the business and science of medicine, often at the exclusion of the sweetness of the physician-patient relationship. The art of medicine does indeed require us to become daring enough to care. This book is a must-read for all medical professionals.
– **Kavitha Chinnaiyan, MD**
Professor of Medicine, Oakland University, Michigan USA
Author of *The Heart of Wellness, Glorious Alchemy,* **and** *Shakti Rising*

A bare-all, honest and lovingly written book that serves as a reminder to all of us of the purpose of medicine. Through the vivid descriptions of many soul-searching experiences, Dr. Bonhoeffer is showing us how the journey of a medical doctor is intertwined with life. This is a journey of love at its core, where passion, service, honesty to oneself and others, humility, devotion, commitment, and intense reflection are necessary complements. Very much like life itself. It takes courage to share one's journey, and Dr. Bonhoeffer does so with grace and elegance.
Flor M. Munoz, MD, MSc
Associate Professor of Pediatrics
Baylor College of Medicine, Houston, Texas

Dare to Care is a compassionate, heartfelt, love-filled narrative about the true vocation and practice of medicine. A much-needed book to be read on this mechanized and corrupt medical model.
– **Carlos Warter, MD, PhD**
Psychiatrist, Guest Lecturer, University of California San Diego

Author of *Recovery of the Sacred, Who Do You Think You Are? The Healing Power of Your Sacred Self,* **and six other books**

Dare to Care is so empowering, so clearly heartfelt, and written with such reverence and seeming unabashed honesty... I would hope that it could be in the eyes, hands, minds, and heart of every student-physician, intern, resident: it was often new and enriching. I will specifically reference the book in my upcoming lectures and workshops.
– **Daniel P. Kohen, MD**
Professor of Pediatrics, University of Minnesota (Retired)
Co-Founder, National Pediatric Hypnosis Training Institute
Co-Author of *Hypnosis and Hypnotherapy With Children*

It would be wise for those entering the practice of medicine as well as those practicing medicine to read *Dare to Care*. When the science, technology, and workload become all-consuming, for many doctors it is easy to lose sight of what we came here for – to awaken and heal oneself and others into Oneness. *Dare to Care* will take you by the hand and compassionately lead you home to your loving nature. I urge you and anyone on the path of awakening to read it.
– **Leonard Laskow, MD**
Guest Lecturer at University of California San Francisco (retired)
Founder of Holoenergetic Healing, Author of *For Giving Love* **and** *Healing with Love*

Dare to Care is a heart-warming reminder of the precious inspirations and human strengths physicians bring with them to their training, and the importance of keeping hold of these, while training and professional life can, if allowed, dampen their glow. This book inspires reflection, trust, and love, and keeps the reader grounded with humanity.

fundamental principle is to engage and establish trust with each person, through deep respect for each individual, and support from a culture that is heart-based. A more scholarly approach might pack in numbers and analyses, but the powerful emotional impact of this uplifting collection would be diluted. These letters are ostensibly directed toward one person, but they are really for all of us.

– **Steven Hirschfeld, MD, PhD**
Professor of Pediatrics, Uniformed Services University of the Health Sciences, Bethesda, Maryland
Captain, United States Public Health Service (retired)

... provides a magic mixture of deeply personal revelations, and stories of children and families whose life experiences taught Prof. Bonhoeffer the wisdom and spirit he so generously shares with us. While both authors speak to Hannah, their words are addressed to those of us who strive to serve others as doctors and other healthcare professionals and seek a way to balance our lives. Humbling, sincere, humane, and genuine, these letters can be used by young and older healthcare professionals as a source of daily wisdom, comfort, and motivation. I hope you enjoy it as much as I did.

– **John van den Anker, MD, PhD**
Eckenstein-Geigy Distinguished Professor of Pediatric Pharmacology
University of Basel, Childrens' Hospital, Switzerland

Dare to Care comes from a deep heart that knows that caring and compassionate interaction is the underpinning of healing and of connection where our heart's intuitive guidance combines with our mind's knowledge to best serve others. Whether doctor, coach, counselor, friend, parent, or

spouse, compassionate care is a gift to each other and our own well-being.
— **Deb Rozman, PhD**
Co-CEO HeartMath Inc., Boulder Creek, Colorado

Not only a great read for patients, but also a must-read for medical professionals who want to keep their faith or regain it. *Dare to Care* highlights the initial motivation of health care professionals: a heartfelt sense of love and meaning which should not be sacrificed on the altar of technical knowledge and scientific protocol. To the contrary, science may be complemented by a heart-based approach serving as an inner guide to deeper wisdom. Where science reaches its limits, both physician and client deserve to enter a resonant field, access fresh insight, and find deep meaning.
— **Bence Ganti, MA**
Clinical psychologist, Hungary
Founder, Integral Academy and the Integral European Conferences

Deeply moving, the authors invite health care professionals to explore our ability to change patterns of belief and behavior in our continued quest toward improving our effectiveness. Reading *Dare to Care* is an enjoyable and heartwarming journey of well-guided neuroplastic growth and realignment on the path or true healing. I highly recommend this wonderful book to curious doctors, nurses, and therapists alike.
— **Anat Baniel**
Clinical Psychologist
Founder of Anat Baniel Method® and NeuroMovement®

In a time of COVID, this book offers a gentle wisdom that quietly empowers the reader to understand that, in the end, it is simple human goodness that endures and it is the heart that generates healing. It thereby points to a more refined human future.

– **Jim Garrison PhD**
Founder / President, Ubiquity University

Welcome

To the World of Heart-Based Medicine

DARE TO CARE

*How to Survive and Thrive in
Today's Medical World*

Dr. Jan Bonhoeffer

Arjuna Ardagh

Dare to Care
Copyright © 2020 by Dr. Jan Bonhoeffer and Arjuna Ardagh

Published by:
Heart-Based Medicine Foundation
Güterstrasse 154
4053 Basel
Switzerland

heartbasedmedicine.org

ISBN 978-0-578-80923-6

For Jessica
in gratitude for her endless patience.

Both authors bow
in deep respect.

Table of Contents

Foreword _____ xii

Your Sparkling Eyes _____ 1

Remember Why You Came _____ 16

You Just Know _____ 32

Listen to Your Patients _____ 46

You are Treating People, Not Conditions _____ 64

Taking Care of Yourself is Fundamental _____ 81

Trust Resonance _____ 102

Don't be Afraid to Break the Rules _____ 118

Question "Normal" _____ 138

Dare to Care _____ 153

Create Loving Relationships _____ 174

Believe in Healing Potential _____ 192

Set the Tone for the Day _____ 208

Learn from Mistakes _____ 221

Choose Your Role Models _____ 234

Connect With the Infinite _____ 250

Conclusion _____ 269

Afterword _____ 276

Acknowledgements _____ 281

"In times of rapid change the learners will inherit the earth, while the knowers will find themselves beautifully equipped to deal with a world that no longer exists."

~ Eric Hoffer

Foreword

By Srini Pillay, M.D.

Associate Professor of Psychiatry, Harvard Medical School

When I entered my residency program at Harvard Medical School, I was an eager beaver, wanting to lap up all the information I could, cure all of the patients who came my way, and impress all of my teachers with my dedication, pursuit of knowledge, and the immense love that I felt in my heart for what people are. As if unleashed upon this new and prestigious world, I threw myself into every second with reckless abandon, wondering why my heart was so touched by the laughing manic patient, why I simply could not stop reading about the brain after 36 hours of being on call, and how fortunate I was to be given the privilege of being taught by such loving and thoughtful teachers.

Then, came the day of reckoning — my very first assessment. I knew in my mind that I had crushed this... that there was no way in the world I would not hear pomp and praise come my way like trays of luscious fruit fit for a king. But boy, was I in for a rude shock!

To make a long story short, my beloved teachers lauded my knowledge, efforts, dedication, and heart. "But," they said, "we are worried about you."

"Worried?" I said, befuddled and gazing at falling stars as if someone had punched me in the stomach. "Yes," they replied. "We don't see you sitting on the park benches with your colleagues. You attend 100 percent of your didactics — which shows no discernment. And you never play hooky by swimming with some of them at Walden Pond."

"You see," they explained. "You came to Harvard to be educated to be the best doctor you could ever be — not to acquire knowledge. And education — true education — means that you should build time in your life to reflect, to ponder, to heal yourself, and to allow your thoughts to congeal into higher forms of intuition, insights, and caring. At the rate you're going, you'll burn out five years after graduating."

This feedback was hard to swallow, but being a dedicated student, and someone who understood love even when it was delivered as a bitter pill, I immediately took their words to heart. And when I did, the love and excitement that comes from contact with a creative world and unitary consciousness infused my thirst for knowledge with an undying desire to heal — a desire that has luckily escaped the swords of the cynical.

Dare to Care is a book about the magic of medicine and life. It is about a love affair between doctor and patient that has gone wrong. It is all about how, as patients, we long for caring and connection when we are ill, and how doctors who come to this profession to be Casanovas of consciousness often leave feeling drained and diluted as human beings because they forget who they are. And in this book, the authors play Cupid between doctor and patient so that they may rekindle this special love again.

Love comes from an experience of being whole. Biology teaches us about the various components of the whole, so that we may rejoice in the delicate ways in which serotonin bathes neurons, or how neurons kindle to fire and fill us with meaning, or the myriad feelings that can travel from the gut to the brain and back. These are now all irrefutable and observable facts. Yet perhaps one that rises above them all is the indelible connection between the heart and the brain.

Always writing love letters to each other, the connection between these organs is a physiologic harmony that nurtures the body and all who come into contact with it. And in this book, you will be reminded that this is who you are, and it is what you have been looking for in any doctor you have sought.

I say this, knowing that I am still a knowledge warrior, looking for the next big conquest in understanding, reading science voraciously so as to impart whatever I can to my patients as they try to find themselves in our connection. Like most doctors, I am dazzled by the lights of paradox that come our way. "Eat LDL cholesterol and you will have a heart that is clogged and spluttering," some studies say... until you read the nineteen studies that will tell you that there is no relationship between cholesterol and dying, or, in fact, the very opposite of what you thought. "Eat more LDL cholesterol and you're less likely to die" reports the *British Medical Journal*. And the *American Journal of Cardiology* concurs — when you have higher LDL cholesterol, you'll be less likely to die from a heart attack.

"What?" I hope you're asking. Yes, these are the paradoxes that doctors have to deal with on a daily basis. So you can hardly blame them for politicking their way to opinions about chloroquine for COVID-19, or for preferring the keto diet over the Mediterranean diet because of their personal biases, for instance. If you look long and hard enough, you'll always find ways to support whatever you think.

It's not just that medicine is a dubious and somewhat mind-boggling science, though Marcia Angell, respected scientist and former editor of the *New England Journal of Medicine,* had an even darker view. She said, "It is simply no longer possible to believe much of the clinical research that is published, or to rely on the judgment of trusted physicians or authoritative medical guidelines. I take no pleasure in this conclusion, which I reached slowly and reluctantly over my two decades as an editor of *The New England Journal of Medicine.*" Indeed, Richard Horton, editor of *The Lancet,* also wrote that "The case against science is straightforward: much of the scientific literature, perhaps half, may simply be untrue."

These proclamations may make one instantly turn against medicine, but *Dare to Care* does exactly the opposite. In recognizing medicine's cancer of corruption, it prescribes a formula to join a new bandwidth of caring, intuition, holism, and love, to ride the exceptional waves of being alive to live beyond the norm.

To the up to 80 percent or more of physicians who have been burned out (or hopefully recognize this in themselves), this book is a refreshing reminder of your highest self. And to any patient who still wishes to bathe in the many balms that biology has to offer, it is a glorious gift to give to any physician who is caught in this disastrous maelstrom of confusion. Much recent scientific research has shown that the key to higher intelligence resides in brain entropy. The infinite connection to the self and the world that this book provides is a door to a cataclysm that will rejuvenate any caring heart that is worn, weary, or wanting for a better life.

— **Dr. Srini Pillay**
  Boston, September 2020

Chapter One
Your Sparkling Eyes

My beloved Hannah,

As your godfather, I often think of you with love. I think about your future, about where your life is heading, where you want to go, and how I can best support you in your mission.

You are such a rare flower, such a beautiful expression of this unbelievable life. You are so calm, humorous, and gentle; you have a clear presence and a sharp mind. What strikes me most is the openness of your heart. You have such an infectious, radiant love that everyone around you can feel. Your eyes are full of fire, and love, and curiosity.

I am inspired by your decision to dedicate your life to caring for others. As you know, your father and I were medical students together, and we have both spent our lives in the medical profession. I have spent the last twenty years caring for children and their families. I am overjoyed to welcome you to this path. Your natural loving presence and open heart remind me of the essence of what we are all doing. It is what puts the "care" in healthcare. As your godfather, I am here to support you in every way I can.

*

I remember well the moment when you told me that you wanted to study medicine. We were at the farm, where I was living at the time. You told me that you wanted to become a paramedic, and asked me about the first steps; you knew that it was how I got started myself. You asked me what books to read, and how to prepare. We sat out on the grass, in the sunshine, and talked about what it means to help people who are in dire straits. We talked about the rough parts of all this: we come into people's homes, we see accidents, we see violence, we see suffering; we see it all firsthand in the environment where people are living.

Sitting together in the sunshine, we deeply explored if this was what you really wanted. I can remember the look in your eyes: you were on fire. You passionately wanted to be there for people, to help them, to offer your love and care — which is very real in you. We both knew that you would need to learn the tricks of the trade: how to rescue people from dangerous situations, and how to offer physical support when their bodies are hurt.

I remember well that look in your eyes; I call it the "inner spark." That is what gets us all going and moving in the right direction. It helps us in difficult times, moves us along when we are writing exams, or in the many stressful situations we face as students. That spark has vision, it carries an inner clarity. It is this inner light that carries us through all these situations.

Now that you are moving from being a student to being a resident in a hospital, there will be more and more of these stressful situations. That is why it is so important to notice and foster this light. It is like a little flame that needs to be kindled and nurtured.

After more than twenty years of medical practice, I have to admit that I have all too often forgotten about this light, and dismissed it in the name of science and objectivity. There have been times when I felt that my life as a doctor was reduced to the upper five centimeters of my body. I was only concerned with ideas, with knowledge to be acquired, and analyzed, and distributed. This is how our inner spark can get eclipsed. I had to learn this the hard way.

As I look back, having attended to so many children and families and having had the opportunity to look inside myself, I now know that all this knowledge is just a small part of what is really important to the people we are serving. It is also only a small part of what is important to me, as a doctor, in my desire to enable real healing in people.

*

Hannah, my dear, give me a few minutes of your time. Let me tell you a little about what has moved me deeply in the last years: not only as a doctor, but also as your friend and godfather.

As you know, I studied medicine — just as you did — and I also became a resident — as you are now, and I continued to pursue a medical career along exactly the lines of all I had learned. I have deeply appreciated everything I have learned from my teachers, as I am sure you also appreciate everything you have learned in your studies. There is so much information to take in, so much to learn, and so much to discover about the body. It is an endless playing field. Going down this route has clearly been helpful beyond measure.

A few years ago, however, I started to realize that it was as if I had been going to the gym, but only lifting weights with my right arm. The left arm was not being exercised at all. Let me explain.

When I went to medical school, I was highly motivated by the joy of learning: the endless playground of studying life, studying the human body. I became fascinated by how the complex human being works, and how we can help. Now, as a university professor, I have become knowledgeable, to some degree, and I can share that knowledge with young doctors like you.

But what matters the most, dear Hannah, is not all that accumulated knowledge. That is why I am writing this letter to you today. Although it was intriguing and interesting, it was never what mattered most for me. You can imagine: in twenty years I have seen many, many patients. It was hardly ever the knowledge that mattered most to them either. Everything I learned in medical school, everything I have been taught, everything I have talked about, everything I have tried to absorb and get on top of, it was all important, it all had value, but it was not the most important part of being a doctor.

No, not by far.

Hannah, whenever I look into your innocent eyes, I believe that I can see what really matters to you, and I resonate deeply with what I see there. The fire I recognize in your eyes expresses what matters the most to you, to me, and to more or less everyone who goes into healthcare.

All the knowledge we have accumulated has its place, but only in the much bigger landscape of healing that is nourished not by academic learning, but by what we each bring to healthcare as an authentic, dedicated, vulnerable, and caring human being.

You, Hannah, you. Who you are. That is the real gift.

You can help people with what you have in your mind, but your heart is the vehicle of real healing. It is contained in who you are as a being, and it is expressed in how you show up, and how authentically you make yourself available for your patients. It reveals itself in how deeply you are engaged with them. It is affected by how sincerely you take responsibility for your own well-being, and then it overflows into how you truly care for your patients.

It is the very essence of who you are, and how you nurture yourself, that your success as a healer depends.

Your effectiveness as a real facilitator of health rests only in part on what you have learned. The much bigger part depends on whether you allow yourself to fully open your heart and whether you allow yourself to be fully available for the people you attend to.

*

Do you remember the first time you looked into a microscope, and marveled at the miracle of life itself? Do you remember the moment when you saw this whole new world of tissues, and cells, and how they work and connect with each other? Can you remember that moment? I can clearly remember the moment when the mystery of life opened up for me through science. It was the first time I looked into a microscope and saw a living cell. I have fallen in love with understanding what I had a glimpse off on that day. I went into research to understand it all more. I've written over a hundred research papers, and read countless books. I've been to more conferences that I can remember, always seeking the latest and the best that can be known.

In exactly the same way, there have been moments — just like looking into that microscope — when another mystery has also opened up for me. These are the moments when there is more to healing than scientific knowledge. At school, during clinical training and research, you learn to look at the body from the outside, to describe it and understand it. But whenever I remember to look into this different microscope, this inward microscope, I remember the fundamental importance of how we feel inside ourselves, how alive we feel, and how we each experience our own lives. This other kind of discovery is very different from anything taught in medical school.

I often remember a specific moment, at five or six years old, when I sat in my mother's lap. I was overtaken by a mysterious peace. I felt infinite, connected with everything. That was not a moment that required any medical knowledge, but it was an initiation into the core of true healing. Much later, I traveled to India to do an internship in a hospital. One morning I woke up early. I was sitting quietly on the veranda looking at the river flowing by. Then, suddenly, there was only the river, and the cup of tea, but I was not there anymore as a separate entity. Once again, that moment did not involve any diagnostic tests, or charts, or prescriptions, but it was a moment of dropping into the essence of real healing.

Throughout my life, there have been so many little signs like this along the road. Often, they are nothing special or dramatic, not an extravagant fireworks display. These moments are just little signs tucked away into the fabric of daily life that remind us of what is really important. The more knowledgeable I became, and the more I advanced in my profession, the more I learned to cease paying attention to those signs, and then to dismiss them.

As you went through medical school, and now as you begin your residency, I already see how it is changing you. In many ways, it has been wonderful for you to get trained and to become a safe and competent young doctor. But I can also see your temptation to begin to objectify patients, and this is when the gradual slippery slope of missing those signs begins.

That, dear Hannah, is why I am writing these letters for you.

*

Several years ago, after I had gone pretty far down the rabbit hole of ignoring those reminders and listening only to the voice of scientific knowledge, I heard about a man who has a reputation for stirring things up, and asking a lot of challenging questions. Once I met him, I quickly realized that he is quite uncompromising. I entered into a coaching relationship with this man, with the intention of getting back on track.

Working with him was sometimes gratifying and nourishing, and often confronting and uncomfortable. By slowing down and focusing on my life within the container of this kind of support, I slowly came face to face with my own dishonesty, with myself and with other people, with my narcissism and selfishness, and with my arrogance as an experienced doctor. I thought I was some great guy who could make no mistakes in any area of my life, simply because I had the credentials.

I started out in this coaching relationship to focus on my marriage. Things had gone really downhill. I was making so many mistakes, and being so insensitive as a husband. I recognized that I had lost alignment with myself, with my heart, and it was affecting everything in my life. Everything had become disconnected from the purity and innocence that I once had as a young doctor. Although I was writing prescriptions all day for how other people could get well, I had completely forgotten how to take care of myself, the carer, and my loved ones. This new commitment allowed me to remember how to restore energy and well-being within myself.

Working with a coach in this way also helped me realize that my work as a vaccine-safety specialist, working in global health programs including with the

World Health Organization and in many countries, was coming to an end. There was something deeper calling to be expressed through me. In one of our coaching sessions, he guided me through an exercise he had developed twenty-five years before, which he called "The Future Self." It is a kind of vision quest. He guided me to relax deeply, and then to visualize the best possible future I could imagine. I saw a building where people were happily collaborating. I have no idea why, but I saw a simple countryside villa in Tuscany, Italy. People were living there and interacting with each other about love and medicine with passion and joy. This villa seemed to be a global gathering point for people to gather, and to have workshops and trainings. In this vision, it appeared that I was running the place. After this exercise, my coach encouraged me not to pay too much attention to the specifics: not to assume that we must immediately move to Italy. Instead, he encouraged me to pay attention to the flavor of the vision, the atmosphere, and to notice how I felt within this context.

This vision resonated deeply within me. I had already thought a lot about the role of love in medicine for several years. This vision was the point of no return. I knew I had to do it.

I have been working with that same coach consistently ever since. We travelled together into the remote Alps, in the snow, to a cabin completely off the grid, to take many days together in isolation to explore the vision of restoring the Heart to Medicine. We spent a couple of weeks together on an island in Greece. He came several times to work with me in Basel, and I have been many times to work with him in California. We have been working together for a few years now, and this initial vision has become more and more real. Our work included creating a website, shooting many videos, writing articles, and creating an on-line environment. Sometimes it felt like whenever I woke up in the night, there he was, staring me in the face, holding me responsible to make this vision real. Now, I have invited him to co-author this book with me. You will hear his voice later, and hear about some of the useful tools I have learned that we can share with you.

Today there is a global organization built around the vision of heart-based medicine to explore how we can bring the quality of the heart back into the practice of medicine, without in any way discounting or devaluing the important knowledge that can be learned. We have developed an annual conference, we are building a training program for doctors to learn skills that support presence in the heart, and we are writing a much more extensive book together. We have initiated a research track to gather all the data that supports the impact of love on physical healing. We are bringing together some of the best minds in the world who have explored this already.

*

But, my dear Hannah, I simply cannot bear the thought of you having to wait for months or a year till I have finished my longer book and training program, for me to be able to tell you what I really want to tell you. So I have decided to pull out some of the stories and insights from that book as a preview for you, and any other young health care professionals who might be interested.

I wish I had written these letters to you when you started with medical school, but I was not ready then. Now, I feel inspired to pass on to you — with a sense of urgency — the most important principles that can allow you to honor your heart as you begin to move through your residency years.

You have such a brightness, such an innocence, so much pure love living in your heart. To me, as your godfather, it is important that you can treasure who you are and what you have, and that you can continue to kindle it as you move through your residency.

Residency was a very challenging time for me. It was a time of working countless hours, and it was often a time of finding myself in situations that were very overwhelming. I found myself frequently having to compromise my deeper values. You may find yourself starting to switch into survival mode, just to get through it all. You may be tempted to neglect your own body and your own health, to live on coffee and snack food. There may be a temptation to no longer see a multidimensional human being in front of you, but just to focus on making a diagnosis, writing a prescription, and getting the discharge letter out. *There, done.* You may find yourself getting clamped down by the mechanics of things, and by your need to survive it all. You may find yourself willing to sacrifice the natural wisdom of your heart.

And that, my dear Hannah, is why I feel pulled to write these letters for you now. I don't want to see you go through what I went through. I would love to hold your hand for a moment, to look into your eyes, and to tell you a few things that I would love to have known back then. I cannot bear the thought of your innocence being corrupted by people who may have more knowledge than you, but who may have forgotten about the deeper currents of healing, and about natural love.

Your Sparkling Eyes

You have a deep understanding of what is good for people, and what is good for yourself. Your father is my lifelong friend, and a deeply good and healthy man, in every way. I want to support you. I want to be there for you during this time. When you might be tempted to sacrifice your values, either in how you take care of yourself or how you maintain the spirit of taking care of other people, I want you know that I am here. I want to support you in staying true to your values and your initial motivation for becoming a doctor.

Chapter Two
Remember Why You Came

Dear Hannah,

As you go through your residency, with all the long hours and the difficult decisions, the key to keeping the heart open is to remember to stay connected with why you decided to become a doctor in the first place, and to care for people.

Do you remember the moment, the point of no return, when you decided to become a doctor? I can still remember that day when you told me that this is what you wanted, and when you were asking me for advice about how to go about it. I think you were about eighteen at the time. I remember seeing into your passionate, wide-open heart that wanted to explore and embrace the planet and make a difference. Already back then I could sense the purity, innocence, and clarity in your desire to become a doctor. All of that can so easily get clouded by the kind of training you will go through now as a resident, and by the kind of work realities you will be facing.

Hannah, have you heard the parable of the two wolves? An old Cherokee tells his grandson a story that illustrates the battle within each of us.

> *"My boy," he says, "there is a battle between two 'wolves' inside all of us.*
>
> *One wolf is all the things that cause us and others grief: anger, envy, jealousy, sorrow, regret, greed, arrogance, self-pity, guilt, resentment, inferiority, lies, false pride, superiority, and ego.*
>
> *The other wolf is all the things that create a good life: joy, peace, love, hope, serenity, humility, kindness, benevolence, empathy, generosity, truth, compassion, and faith."*
>
> *The grandson listens, thinks for a moment, and then asks: "Which wolf wins?"*
>
> *The elder simply replies, "The one you feed."*

Hannah, you will also have two wolves to feed in these next years of residency. For you, both wolves have something positive, but different, to offer you and to others.

One wolf is the knower in you. That wolf is ravenous for knowledge, for acquiring new skills: it feeds on books and lectures and research.

The other wolf is your passion to care for people. It feeds on compassionate connection with yourself and with others, and it wants to contribute to the world.

You are the one who gets to decide which wolf you feed, and how much. You do not need to choose between them. It is about finding the right balance.

The training at the university requires us to feed the knowledge-management wolf a lot. It is a very hungry wolf, it needs a lot of feeding, and we spend a lot of time gathering enough food for it to eat, and entertaining its endless hunger. But that does not mean that we need to starve the other wolf.

Some people want to feed only the wolf that has love and compassion, and wants to help, but they are not ready to also sharpen their mind, and acquire the knowledge and skills needed to be a highly qualified doctor. I have met other medical students like this: sometimes they dropped out of medical school, and learned massage or other ways to take care of people. But if you take that path, you will not be able to build comprehensive differential diagnoses and treat illnesses like pneumonia, or take out a tumor. You will not be qualified to provide real medical advice or treatment.

On the other hand, if you only feed the knowledge-based wolf, you will simply become a recognizer of patterns and a broker of treatments, not much more than that. You are trained to learn certain things, to label specific sets of signs and symptoms; you have learned what they might mean, what the disease might be called, which kind of pills to prescribe, what kind of surgical interventions to take. These are all ways of recognizing repeating pathologies and remedies.

Many young doctors, and also many patients, have reflected with me over the years that our current system of training doctors is not primarily oriented toward compassion. Medical students touch on it briefly in the class on taking patient history. There is some degree of importance placed on building a relationship with the patient before you ask questions, but mostly, you simply learn the techniques of communication that appear to mimic real compassion, just as a plastic orange might look like a real fruit from a distance. No juice. No nourishment.

When you go to a big store like Walmart in America, the cashier greets you by saying, "Hello, how are you today?" They are trained to say that. Or when you go to a restaurant, the waiter is trained to smile from ear to perfect ear, and to say "Hello, my name is Kim, I will be taking care of you tonight. What can I do for you?" Later the same waiter might ask, "How does everything taste?" But it is empty rhetoric: they have been trained to use that language. Similarly, you can be trained in medical school to mimic the language of real compassion, but you may not be trained to access genuine compassion in your heart. The risk is too great of actually feeling something that could crack the sterile formica veneer of the treatment room.

My hope for you, dear Hannah, my deep prayer for you, is that you will find a way to feed both wolves. I did not do that as much as I had intended, I had no one to hold me accountable to feed both wolves, and it took me twenty years and a coach before I could set this straight. More about that in a moment. One current word for feeding both wolves is "holistic medicine." But this word is often confused with non-conventional medicine, alternative medicine, or adding some kind of "–ology" to conventional medical training.

You become a master of health — for real — only when you explore deeply for yourself what it means to be healthy, what it means to feel alive and energized, what it means to learn to care for your own body, and what it means to lovingly appreciate the diverse expressions of life on this planet.

Like this, you can retain the ability to appreciate and serve the uniqueness of your patients, with all of their gloriously different characteristics, rather than following a protocol based on statistical means and standard deviations. That kind of standardized medicine assumes that everyone is built the same, rather in the same way that every 2008 Honda Civic is built, and can therefore be diagnosed, and repaired, in the same way.

I am writing you these letters simply because they are exactly the letters I wish someone had written to me, when I was at your stage of medical training. Let me tell you now a little bit of how I have found, and lost, and found again my initial motivation.

When I was seven years old, I remember browsing through a folder where my parents stored all their passports and important documents. Giggling at the photos of my mom and dad when they were young, my eyes fell on a tiny leaflet, and I asked my mother what it was. Smiling warmly, she replied, "It's my first-aid certificate." I felt an immediate resonance with this. Even at that age, it woke up my desire to help people feel better; it ignited a spark.

"I want to learn this too!" I declared. My mother was a professional actress, keen to nurture empathy, compassion, and emotional exploration within her young son, so she took me along to the Red Cross ambulance hub the following week.

"My son would like to take a first-aid course. Is there one for kids?" she asked a big, bold man in a white and orange uniform. He was very supportive of my decision but explained that I was a bit too small.

"Why don't you come back when you're about fourteen years old," he suggested. My little world collapsed around my ears. But there was no choice; I would have to be patient.

Meanwhile, my father would spend countless hours satisfying my enquiring mind with science and observation. His favorite question was, "What did you learn from this?" as we took morning strolls together, identifying birds by their songs. Together we would conduct chemical experiments, surprised at our results. As we peered through the microscope and telescope, he would awaken me to the beauty of life's creative expression.

Seven years later, at the ripe old age of fourteen, I signed up for my first-aid course, which eventually led to a paramedic apprenticeship. I was still at school when I completed the full training, so had to spend all my weekends and holidays studying, and even sometimes worked nights during the regular school week. It was a fascinating journey. By that time, with over two thousand hours of experience on the road as a paramedic, I had seen far too many accidents and a great deal of trauma. Although I'd learned many techniques to save lives, there was still a sense of longing inside, a yearning to understand and serve at a deeper level.

As I sat on the deck of the ambulance hub one night, reflecting on our mission the night before and remembering my admiration for the anaesthetist who'd taken charge of the scene, the road ahead became clear. I would become an emergency physician.

The day I signed up for medical school, I strode toward the University, gliding on invisible wings. I felt the sun on my skin and inhaled the crisp morning air like a nourishing breakfast. Entering the building, I steered toward the chancellery like someone who already knew their way. Every cell of my body fizzed and tingled, the leaves in the courtyard dancing in the wind as the morning light bounced off the windows of the long corridor: a feeling I had known previously only from adventure sports. I was twenty-three years young, just out of mandatory military service in

Switzerland, and a new phase of my life was about to begin.

I was following my calling. I was determined to learn everything about the human body, mind, and soul so that I could serve people well.

Once I completed the necessary formalities, signed the right forms, and got my student card, I stood in line to enter a huge room, along with three hundred others who were anxiously also waiting to enter. Everyone was early that day, energized like horses rearing to get out of the stable. Each one was ready to start their own professional life, and for everyone it was a very high energetic moment.

Everyone I spoke to was highly motivated, highly alert, fully present. I looked around and talked with some of the people I would be studying with, and getting to know very well, over the next years. "Where are you from? What is your name? Why are you here?" Everybody wanted to experience something, to contribute something. Everyone was ready, often for the first time, to drive the car of their own lives, to no longer live at home with their parents, to start their adult life. Quickly I discovered that people came with very different motivations.

Thomas was the son of the CEO of a multinational corporation. His early life had trained him to think about power and recognition and influence. He did not want to just become a doctor, he wanted to become a chief medical director, running a big hospital. He wanted to be a powerful person. There were a few others with a similar vision.

Then I remember Nadja. Her parents had immigrated to Switzerland, and she was the first generation to be born here. She wanted to win a Nobel Prize. She saw medical school as the first step to having immense social recognition. When you go to a social gathering, people often ask, "What do you do?" When you can say "I am a doctor," you may win a little extra recognition. There were many students there who thought that they would gain elevated social status by going through this long training.

Franz had been born into a poor family in a rural area of Switzerland. Within a few minutes of speaking with him, he told me that doctors do not have to worry about money. Unlike his father, who drove a delivery van, Franz wanted to always have enough income to support his family.

Peter had always had very low grades in high school. He had just scraped into medical school. His main motivation was to prove to himself, and to his father, that he was actually a smart person, and he could do something significant. I got to know him quite well over the next years, and I saw him time and time again collapsed back into the feeling "I'm not good enough... I'm a bad student... I'm stupid." He went all the way through medical school just to prove that he could do it.

In that first week, I heard that people had all sorts of ideas of why they were there. Maria did not even want to become a doctor. She wanted to study languages and arts, but she had been forced into medical school by the expectations of her parents. They would not allow her to study anything that did not win bread, and was not socially respected.

However, most wanted to heal people, to help people, to make the world a better place: their motivation was compassionate, a call from the heart. Some did not have that motivation right away, but they too found it after a while, as soon as their training involved contact with real people.

With these various motivations, we embarked eagerly together on the long journey of learning, and memorizing all that science knows to date. We used to joke together, and call this the "current state of ignorance," because as fast as we were learning, new things were being discovered and sometimes contradicting what had been taught before.

Only one third of students would pass the exams, two thirds failed or gave up. I was determined to get through. This meant countless hours of study, discussion, debate, and memorizing thousands of pages from a huge stack of medical books.

I remember one lab class in histopathology. We were in pairs, looking into our microscopes, witnessing the beauty and miracle of nature. I felt like a small boy again, filled with awe and joy, and I nudged my neighbor who was equally awestruck. We laughed together with delight at the miracle of it all. The harsh voice of our disgruntled professor blasted through the loudspeaker: "Quiet please, gentlemen. This is not a kindergarten. Some people are trying to study here."

That was one of the many times when my natural enthusiasm died another small death.

During those many years, we learned that the main approach to overcoming diseases was the application of drugs and surgery. There were no courses on how to promote health; in fact, even preventative health measures like vaccines, or the importance of nutrition and clean water, were not taught back than.

There was absolutely no mention of love or compassion on one single day of those five years of study, even though that had been the initial motivation to be there for me, and for many of my fellow students. In fact, during medical school and residency, I learned how not to take care of myself! I learned how to ignore my body's needs, work crazy long hours in stressful situations, and how to perform under tremendous pressure. The understanding was that this was the best way to learn: it was all about the hours on the ward, the number of patients you see, the charts and tests you review. I learned a lot, but at a great price. I am not only talking about the loss of leisure time, or the impact on friendships, or the effect of stress on my health. There is also a huge price paid in losing connection with compassion, with love, with access to our healing hearts. Slowly, day by day, week by week, month by month, that flame of passion to be a healer, to connect with compassion from the heart, was suffocated.

It is my hope, Hannah, in writing these letters to you, that you can keep this flame alive, even as you assimilate all the knowledge you need to become a well-trained doctor. Though it may sound overwhelming, it is not only possible but even enjoyable. Let's take a first simple step:

In the next days or weeks, take a pen and a paper (much better than a keyboard!) and jot down some notes on why you came into medicine.

> *What was you initial motivation?*
> *Where do you want to go with your pursuit of healing?*

Tune into your heart for these answers.

> *What do you feel called to do with patients, now and in the future?*
> *How would you like to see medicine grow and evolve?*
> *What would you like to see as the future of medicine?*

Just now, you still have an innocent, fresh, unclouded perspective. It is truly worth putting this to paper, taking time for it, and exploring it deeply. Perhaps you can write these thoughts in a very special notebook or journal, maybe bound with leather, with a nice strap or buckle.

I would also love for you to find a small object that you can carry with you always like a talisman. You will need to choose and be guided to what that is. We could call that your healer's talisman: something small that you can always treasure. This small object can help you to remember. When you feel worn out, when you have doubts or you feel hopeless or frustrated, when you are with someone who is dying, or you witness any kind of great suffering, you can slip your hand into the pocket of your white coat or your scrubs. Instead of reaching for a coin for the vending machine, you reach for your healing talisman. This may help you to remember your values, to remember why you came; it may help you to relax, to take time alone and to breathe deeply and to refresh yourself from within. It will remind you of what you stand for, what you have dedicated your life to, and what you want to commit to moving forward.

This initial motivation is not something small or transient. It is actually what drives you, and what allows you to stay connected to yourself and your heart.

It is everything.

It is the boat that carries you across the rough waters of difficult times. Whether you are struggling with yourself, or struggling in breaking bad news to a patient, or struggling through difficult journeys with patients, it is this initial motivation that carries you.

As your godfather, I will be here to help you to remember why you came, to encourage you to stay true to your path, and not to become too carried away by all the things you will need to learn, to remember, and to master.

Chapter Three
You Just Know

Dear Hannah,

As you get the freedom and competence to act more independently in the next months and years of residency, you will sometimes have to make critical decisions. Some of them will have massive consequences, and could even determine life or death for others.

You will have to decide whether to give a drug or not, which drug to give, at what dose, when to do everything you can to prolong life, and when to offer someone the opportunity to let go of their life peacefully. There is always the temptation, because of the way you have been trained, to make these kinds of decisions scientifically and empirically — as though there is only one correct answer, and if you just have access to the correct data, you will make the right decision.

When you are called upon to make a decision about the life of someone you are caring for, it is not just another logical conclusion at a node in a decision tree algorithm. These moments have real impact on real people. You will be trained to follow protocol, and to make your decisions based on the best empirical evidence. You will also be trained to recognize when you don't know, and then to seek out the answers in books, online research, medical literature and textbooks, and then perhaps to also ask your attending or consultant specialists who have more experience. All of this is useful, and in fact essential.

However, from time to time you will recognize that there is a quality of intuition, knowing what is right, even when it sometimes seems illogical. There are times when the protocols you learn in medical training will align with your intuition, and there are times when they do not. Sometimes you will hear an inner voice speaking, which may or may not agree with what you have learned in your training. Doctors are trained to label intuition as unscientific and to dismiss this inner voice, rather than listen to it.

This letter I am writing to you today is about this little inner voice. I would love to strengthen it in you, and to encourage you to give it your attention, and to listen.

There are a couple of reasons why this is so important. One is because this little inner voice sits very close to your initial motivation, to the core of why you care; it is a useful reminder of what heartfelt healthcare means. The second reason is that you will very often have to make decisions where you simply do not have the time to think. You will find yourself at a crossroads where life and death are at stake. You will have no time to do the research, to train or educate yourself. You will have to make a decision anyway, in the moment.

This is a resource that you already have within you. It is not something that has to be added to you. No one can teach this to you in medical school. It is a wisdom that is already alive within you; we simply have to make sure that it is sustained, nurtured, and not squashed by your training. It is who you are.

In this letter today I want to encourage you to keep an open channel for this inner voice: to keep your knowledge in your right hand, and your intuition — your inner guidance — in your left hand. I want to encourage you to be aware that there are moments when knowledge can guide you, and there are moments when empirical knowledge can be misleading.

There will be times when you need to know, in a finger snap, what to do, when it is time to save someone's life. There will also be times when you will need to know when it's time to switch off the machine, and when there is nothing more to do. I want to share with you the first time that I witnessed this ability to know, without the need for much evidence.

*

As you know, I started my training as a paramedic when I was sixteen, and I finished the training when I was eighteen. I worked as a paramedic while I was still in school, between eighteen and twenty.

One July night, around 11 p.m., I was in Bavaria in the back of the ambulance. There is a driver, a paramedic, and then there is a third person in training in the back. That was me.

There was a seat along the side, a little desk and drawers with all the things you need for emergency interventions. I was standing behind all this, squeezed in the side door and looking through the window to the driver's cockpit. We were driving through the town at 90 miles an hour.

That night, we had already seen terrible things. First, we were called to a home where a baby had fallen out of his father's arms into a barbecue. The baby was still alive, but very badly burned. You can only begin to imagine how traumatic such a scene is: the baby was severely injured, but also both parents were beside themselves with panic.

From this scene, we were called to a fight at the lakeside. Some men were out on the pier where the cruise ships dock. They were very drunk, and they each held a Weissbier beer glass, which is tall and thin. One of these men became very angry with another man; he knocked his glass against the wooden railing of the pier, and used the remaining stem of the glass as a weapon. By the time we arrived, one man's throat was completely cut open, as though with a razor. The carotid artery had been completely severed, and blood was pulsing out, spraying all over the ground. He was unconscious; each of us took an arm and inserted the largest needles. We gave him liters of infusions within a few minutes. That was the twelfth of the calls we had responded to that evening. We dropped the patient off at the hospital, barely stable, and we were ready to go home. That was when we got another call to drive to

Andechs, a monastery on the other side of a very wooded area.

Evidently, some people had been drinking at the monastery, had driven down the road too fast, did not make a bend in the woods and hit a tree. It was a hot and humid night in July, just prior to a thunderstorm. Once again, we drove at 90 miles an hour to this next accident. We were all sweating profusely. I was already completely exhausted at this point: I was still a college student.

When we arrived, the emergency physician was already there, a very experienced doctor. She was a very short woman, slightly obese, with a military-style very short haircut. We were the ones with the equipment. It was the middle of the night, in the middle of the forest, in the pitch dark, and very hard to see. In the distance, I could see the fire engine coming, and the police.

"Bring the response bag, the monitor, and the ventilator," the driver instructed. I unhooked these three heavy things, and carried them over to the scene of the accident. The emergency physician was attending to the driver.

"There's a girl higher up on the roadside," she barked at me, without even looking up. "Go and attend to her." By now a lot of emergency vehicles had arrived, blue lights flashing. It was hard to see. Everything was very bright, then suddenly pitch black. I took the flashlight, and faintly I could see the figure of an adolescent girl. Her body was completely distorted; the face was no longer recognizable at first sight, full of blood, and totally cut open. One arm was turned upward in a completely unnatural posture. Her belly was cut open, so you could see the intestines. Then I realized: it was a girl from my school. I didn't know her very well, but I saw her every day.

At this point, we had no idea if she was alive or dead. None of this looked very compatible with life, but we rushed to do all we could. At first, it seemed there might be signs of life, so we started with CPR, intubation, ventilation, fluids, drugs, monitoring — the works. For about half an hour, we did everything we could to try to get her back. This was heavy physical work; we were all profusely sweating.

The emergency physician had been attending to the others in the car; she came over suddenly to where we were working.

"Okay... stop," she barked at us.

That was all she said. I was completely shocked. This was not just a random statistic, this was a girl of about my age, who went to my school. Thoughts flew through my head in panic. "You've got to be... What on earth... Who on earth are you...?"

That emergency physician saw my bewilderment, my shock. She was experienced enough to realize what was happening for me.

"What is going on with you, young man?" she asked.

I could not utter a word. I was completely and totally overwhelmed by the horror I was experiencing. She gave instructions quickly to the others, and then she turned to me.

"Come to my car," she said. I followed her. She sat in the driver's seat, and I sat next to her. She turned and looked at me. Suddenly this rough, military woman became very soft. She became very loving and motherly.

"What happened to you?" she asked me, softly.

Now I could speak again. "I'm shocked... how could you... on what grounds... who are you to make this decision... this was a girl I knew. We had just been working on her for half an hour... it seemed like there still might be some hope to bring her back... you just came over... took the briefest glance... made a decision to end her life. How is that possible?"

Briefly, she explained her rationale. I became still. I couldn't follow with my brain, but it equally made no sense to my heart. How was it possible to make such a decision about another human being?

Then she said, "You know, Jan, it is the strangest thing. I have been doing this job now for more than thirty years. I've seen a lot. You are just starting. And sometimes... you just know."

Somehow, the way she said those words, the calm, sad confidence with which she spoke, let me know that she was right. She knew it was pointless, and she was not afraid to make the decision.

I often think back to that moment, Hannah. With everything I have learned in the intervening thirty years, I can only now fully understand that she made the right decision. At the time I could not see it: I did not have the knowledge or the experience.

This was a powerful moment for me. With all of her decades of training and experience, this woman had developed the ability to listen to her intuition, and to know immediately what to do, without letting it get drowned out by protocol and data.

Even as you begin this journey, as you are still accumulating knowledge and experience, you will sometimes still need to rely upon the things that you just know.

I mentioned to you in a previous letter that sometimes I will pass you over to Arjuna. As a coach with more than thirty years experience of supporting people to be the very best version of themselves, he has a few tricks up his sleeve. He has shared a lot of them with me, and now he will share some with you too.

*

Hi, Hannah. Here are a few tips that you can use to access and listen to that inner voice that Jan has talked about here.

Tune into your breastbone

Here is a valuable tool I learned from my colleague Sonia Choquette, an internationally recognized expert on developing intuition. When you are faced with a tough decision, alongside the more empirical analytical data available to you, bring your awareness to your breastbone, or your sternum. Is it lifting upward, toward the sky, in a way that allows you to breathe more easily? Or is it pushing down, and contracted?

Sonia Choquette tells us that the sternum is something like a little antenna which allows you to access knowing beyond thinking. When it feels heavy and pushed down, it can indicate that you are intuitively not feeling completely okay about something. Something is off. When your sternum feels lifted up and light, even when it involves a decision to switch off life support, it may indicate that your intuition is telling you that it is the right thing to do. When your sternum lifts in this way, you have the feeling of holding your head up high, your torso lifts.

Even as I write this, I can hear the voice of the skeptic, saying something along the lines of "Oh, great, so here's this doctor from Switzerland advising his goddaughter to listen to some California quack telling her to make all her medical decisions on how she feels in her sternum. Good luck with that!" Of course, that is not what we are saying here. You will have access to all the data, you will have all your training, and you have support. But when you also need to add the important element of what feels right and good and true, this may serve you as it served many others.

Ask others

There is also another way to feel more confident about what is the right thing to do in any situation. If it feels right to you, it will probably feel right to others as well. As you develop your capacity to listen to your intuition, you can speak with others who are also tuned into their intuition. This may not simply be a question of asking everyone who has read the same textbook, and who has the same training as you, because they will probably not answer from intuition, but from what they have read. You can scan the environment to see who may be most connected to what feels right.

*

Here is Jan again. When I want to get support for my intuition, I have often turned to a very senior doctor, who has been around for a long time, and is even about to retire. Such a doctor has often been through enough that they have learned through the school of hard knocks, and such a doctor may have intuitive knowledge that eclipses what seems logically true. This may sometimes drive you nuts. For sure, it drove me nuts at the time. Doctors in their prime years will want to train you with precise knowledge and information. The older doctors don't adhere to the guidelines as much. They can be a little more rebellious. That is because they are following them less, and intuiting more. By aligning your own intuition with that of an older doctor, rather than comparing their actions with what you have learned, you will have the benefit of the knowledge you get from medical school combined with the wisdom of the heart.

I have also found that the nurses are often very aligned with their intuition. Some people will encourage you to think of nurses as simply your support team: your assistants. You make the decisions, they carry out your decisions. As you are starting out, however, most of the nurses will have more experience than you. Nurses have not had to absorb quite as much data and knowledge as the doctors, and hence they may have a better capacity to access intuition. They also spend more time at the patient's bedside. When you have a strong intuition of what is right or not right, ask the nurse how he or she feels about it. This has almost always paid off for me, as well as the patients I cared for.

There are also others in the hospital room who are most deeply affected by your decisions: the parents of a child, or the family members who may soon be bereaved if things don't go well. Those close to the patient will have their fears, their feelings of hopelessness and powerlessness, which can cloud intuition. If you learn to respect them, to ask them in a calm way to feel what intuitively feels right, you will discover if it aligns with what also feels right to you.

Finally, you can ask the most important person in this equation: your patient. Depending on their age and condition, you may be able to ask what feels right or not right, what feels true or not true, and see how it aligns with your own intuition. Sometimes, your patient's intuition may completely fly in the face of science and empirical results, and then you have to take it with a pinch of salt. When the data and the tests are ambiguous, and when you have a strong intuitive sense of what is going on, you can see if that aligns with the patient's intuition as well.

Some of the most valuable moments in my clinical life working with patients were when I noticed that the data, or even my own intuition, was not connected with the patient's intuition. Then I have learned to stop, not to push through with my agenda, but to hold off for a moment, to recalibrate, and to be curious why our different intuitions about the next right thing were not aligned. Taking time for this has frequently saved hours and weeks afterwards, and then set the healing process in the right direction.

Chapter Four
Listen to Your Patients

Dear Hannah,

For as long as we can remember, medicine has been dominated by and practiced by men. It has created a certain kind of masculine culture. The doctor is the one with all the answers. He knows what is wrong, he knows the solution, and the intended outcome. The patient is something like an insect lying on its back, wiggling its legs helplessly in the air, passively being treated, and very vulnerable.

The culture is shifting as more women come into medicine. But the system is still skewed toward seeing the doctor as an expert. An expert is someone who has the role, in any interaction, of disseminating their expertise, talking a lot, having all the answers, and benevolently dispensing their wisdom to others.

I have discovered, sometimes painfully, that this often serves the identity of the doctor more than the patient.

Recently I have developed a friendship with the relationship expert John Gray, who wrote *Men Are from Mars, Women Are from Venus.* He recognizes the biochemical, and particularly the hormonal, differences between men and women. John pointed out to me that when a woman is not feeling good, often what helps the most, more than giving advice or fixing problems, is for someone to simply listen. When someone simply listens, is deeply curious, it bestows respect. It gives attention and curiosity, which are all qualities very close to the wisdom of the heart, qualities close to love. Simply being listened to in this way stimulates the release of oxytocin into the bloodstream, which, particularly for a woman, reduces stress.

Men, on the other hand, run more on higher levels of testosterone. As you know, this is a hormone associated with solving problems, pushing through difficulties, and getting things done. So, as long as medicine has been dominated by men, the emphasis came from this testosterone-influenced viewpoint. *"Win the battle with cancer... Kill the germs... We will fight this together... What are your health goals...?"* As I have become aware of this, I have been listening to the language my colleagues use more closely. Male doctors tend to use predominantly military and forceful metaphors to describe illness and healing. Those in positions of leadership are called "officers," like the chief executive and chief medical officers.

The alternative is not to adopt different metaphors in the attempt to explain things to the patient, but to do the opposite: to learn to listen deeply and compassionately.

In medical school, you learn about listening when training in how to take patient history. This is a very specific way of asking questions with a defined aim: to filter out signs and symptoms, to recognize patterns, and then to give them a diagnostic label. That style of listening serves to arrive efficiently at a diagnosis, which is also often what the patient expects you to do. But, dear Hannah, you may discover that there is something missing in this way of listening. To discover this for yourself, you have to experiment with another approach.

In another of my letters I will talk with you about creating "resonance." The way that we listen is one of the most powerful ways to create resonance. When you connect with your patient, and listen deeply, listen actively, when you listen deeper than the story that they are telling you, you will hear things you would miss with the conventional approach. Getting important information from people does not only depend on the questions you ask, it also depends on the attitude you bring to the listening. Changing your attitude around listening not only changes the answers you will receive, but it allows the other person to feel more comfortable, more relaxed, more trusting, and more open.

When taking a patient history, I have many times diverted this possibility by efficiently and effectively whizzing down the differential diagnostic algorithms. This is how I was trained, and it is probably how you will be trained too. Once I became aware of it, it took me quite some time to let go of this habit, and to learn to listen to my patient with no intention to figure out a diagnosis, but just with the pure intention to learn, and listen, and hear what is really important to that person.

In medical school, they will tell you that the first question you ask is an open question: "What brings you to the hospital today? Why are you here?" Then you are trained to pause and listen. But what typically happens when you are pressed for time, is that you listen until you get the first clue, and then the cogs start turning in your brain, and you quickly go down the rabbit hole of diagnostic algorithms.

In order to keep your heart open and your compassion alive, it is immensely valuable to know how to listen in a way that creates deeper resonance.

*

Let me tell you the story of Tina.

When Tina came to my office with her mother for the first time, I came out to collect them in the crowded waiting room. "Tina Rossi, please," I called out, loudly. I was looking for a fourteen-year-old girl in the crowd. When she stood up, I saw a very tall and slim girl, with short blonde hair and a pale complexion. She lifted herself out of the chair as if it was against her deeper intentions. She was wearing outdoor sporty kind of clothes, light track shoes, and she moved slowly toward me in small steps with her upper body slightly bent forward, her shoulders slumped, and her head turned toward the floor. She was followed by her mother, who had longer gray hair, and was dressed in flowing, fashionable French clothes. Her mother looked at me with confidence as she said, "Good morning, Dr. Bonhoeffer," and shook my hand warmly.

As we sat down in my office together, all of us around the same small round table, I greeted them. "Welcome, Tina; welcome, Mrs. Rossi."

"Thank you, we are glad to be here. We were referred to you by Dr. Romano, our family pediatrician where we were living previously. He recommended that we see you here in this district we moved to. Tina has a lot of complaints, and we really need to make progress." Mrs. Rossi spoke with an exhausted tone in her voice.

"Tina, tell me. What is bothering you?" After the urgency expressed in her mother's voice, I expected a similarly urgent response from the teenager. Instead, it took almost a minute for her to answer, as Tina looked down to the floor between her knees, her head drooping. "I don't know, there's so much," she quietly muttered.

I paused, waiting for her to continue. Over the next forty-five minutes, between Tina and her mother speaking, I learned about her splitting headaches, the unremitting heartburn she had experienced for the last six months, her stomachache that had not let up for almost a year, her loss of appetite and sense of being overweight despite actually losing weight, her lower back pain, the pain in her right knee and left ankle. She told me about the dry red itchy skin in her elbows and knees, and how it kept getting worse. She had trouble concentrating at school, her homework took her mostly late into the night, and then she could not fall asleep easily, and woke up in the morning with anxiety, as if run over by a truck.

I was curious to know if she ever had times when she felt better. She told me that she loved to dress in rugged outdoor clothing, and spent most of her weekends in nature, out in the mountains, with a group of boys camping and watching birds.

"Thank you, Tina," I said. "This is really a lot of great information. I feel we need more time to get to the bottom of this than the usual office visit. It would be very good for us to see each other again, so we can help you feel better." They both nodded. "May I suggest that we find an appointment in the next few days where I will examine you thoroughly, and we can determine if we need any lab tests? Then we can add a third appointment, where we can review all the results and make a plan on how we can meet your needs. How would that work for you?"

We all agreed, and she left with a slightly more energized disposition, as she walked toward the reception desk to arrange for the next appointment.

When I saw her the next time, Tina's body posture had not changed. "How are you today, Tina?" I asked. She shrugged her shoulders, suggesting that nothing had improved since our last appointment. We went through an extensive physical examination, in the presence of her mother. It revealed nothing abnormal, except her eczema. I thanked her for her for permission to examine her, and we discussed my proposed lab tests.

"I see here that you are taking eight medications. There is nothing wrong with any of them, but I'm not exactly sure whether you really need them just now, and how they really modify what is going on in your body. Given how long you have been struggling already, I would like to propose stopping all of them, and just keeping the painkillers in reserve, if you really need them. What do you think about that idea?"

Tina nodded enthusiastically, and her mother confirmed. They both breathed a sigh of relief...

At the end of the second consultation, I had a hunch that the lab work would probably not shed any additional light on what we would need to get to the bottom of this. I followed the teenager and her mother to the reception desk. "Julia, would you be kind enough to find an appointment for us at the end of the day, one day this week, to discuss the lab results. We may need some extra time to discuss things more deeply."

The third time she came in, I went to collect them in the waiting room. They were the last ones there. They both stood up quickly, as if nervous. We sat down together at the same little round table in my office, and I opened the conversation. "All the lab results came back normal, Tina." She shrugged her shoulders, as if she had already anticipated this. But her nervousness did not settle.

"Tina, we only know each other for about two hours in total, but you came to seek my help. Honestly, I feel that you know something that I do not yet know, something that might explain a lot of your suffering. Is that possible?

After a long pause, looking at the floor, she looked at her mother, who opened her eyes wide as if to encourage Tina to say something that her mother already knew. Then tears started rolling down Tina's cheeks and she whispered, "Yes." She looked at me, she looked back at the floor, she looked at me, she looked at the floor. And then, very quietly and very slowly, she spoke.

"I feel like... like... like... a man... in a woman's body. Nothing really fits. It all hurts. This is not my body. And yet sometimes it is. I feel ashamed. I don't know what to do about any of this."

I moved forward and held her hand. For five minutes, no one said a word.

As her crying settled a little, I continued to hold her hand, and to give her my full attention. "Congratulations," I said. "I am so proud of you! You just took a tremendous step."

She started to collect herself. I gave her a tissue. She straightened up in her seat, wiped her swollen eyes, and blew her nose with great determination. "Thank you for your trust in me, and for sharing all this," I continued. "You have just opened a gate for yourself to walk through."

She sat up more straight in the chair, and took a deep breath. She looked straight into me, with a penetrating gaze. She filled her chest. The position of her feet changed, so they were firmly on the floor. All this was as if to say with her body: "Here I am. See me. I am a young man."

"How do you feel now?" I asked.

"Relieved," she sighed. Her voice sounded deeper, more confident.

"We are on this journey now together," I asserted. "We can build a team to help us learn more, and to find the best route for you moving forward. But before we even take any action, I wonder if you have a hunch as to how many of the complaints you mentioned to me in our first meeting have to do with you feeling like you are a man in a female body?"

Now, for the first time in all of our interactions, she did not hesitate for a moment. Her voice was confident, calm and clear. "All of them, Dr. Bonhoeffer. It is all part of the same thing."

Every cell in my body agreed, as I listened to her. If I had followed the diagnostic training that was so familiar to me, my initial list of suspected diagnoses would include chronic gastritis, juvenile arthritis, atopic dermatitis, anorexia, and many more. My list of extensive diagnostics would have included tons of lab tests, a brain MRI, gastroscopy, and many more. My list of treatment options would have included antacids, anti-inflammatories, antibiotics, and more. I would have followed all of that if I had not listened, without aiming to make a textbook diagnosis.

"It seems to me that it is still a good idea to listen to your body, and to everything that you feel. How about if we take a gentle approach, inviting your body to realign with this new perspective?"

Now, for the first time in all three of our meetings, a broad smile crept across her face. His face. She was grinning at me. He was grinning at me.

"If you had a wish, if it was up to you, what would be the best next step?"

Once again, the reply came without any hesitation, with confidence from the belly. "Drop school for a few days. Eat lightly. Rest most of the day. Drink tea. Do nice things that I enjoy."

And so it was agreed.

I wrote a note for the school, suggesting that Tina needed to rest a lot, and take walks in nature. I recommended her to lie down every morning and every evening for 15 minutes, with a large cup of chamomile infusion, while gently massaging the belly with a clover ointment to relieve the abdominal symptoms. I asked Tina to get hold of an empty notebook, to sketch thoughts and feelings as they arose. I also suggested to take six soothing massages, and a set of physical therapy sessions focusing on

Feldenkrais awareness through movement exercises, which would allow a new style of being in the body to develop.

I was struck by Tina's body language as I proposed all of this. The whole body became more flexible, like it was being inhabited more. She held her hand over her heart for a moment, and looked at me with steady eyes.

"I am looking forward to learning a lot together with you in the weeks to come," I said, as we closed the appointment.

As they left the consulting room, I took a minute to reflect, and to reset myself prior to going home to my family for the evening. Tina taught me a powerful lesson. Recognizing the patterns of disease too quickly, identifying myself as a respected professional applying my knowledge by generating a long list of diagnoses, and then offering an immediate barrage of drugs to relieve the signs and symptoms might not be as helpful as taking more time to build a sincere heart-opening relationship, listening more deeply, and being guided by the patient's own assessments and sense of direction toward greater health. Only then could I offer her some of what I know, both from medical training and my experience from assisting thousands of families. By listening deeply, we were able to radically change the treatment plan, build on her innate healing capacity, and serve her at a level closer to the real cause of her suffering.

I met this patient again, just recently. Now he is a happy, healthy young boy. He did not pursue surgery and hormone therapy so far, and this is still part of his consideration and concern. However, he dresses like a boy. He behaves like a boy, walks like a boy, talks like a boy. He is a boy. He clearly asked me to speak of him in the masculine, as I'm doing now.

That was yet another time when one of my patients kindly taught me to become a better doctor, and a better human being.

As part of my coaching relationship, initially I learned how to listen deeply within the context of my marriage with Jessica. That was the laboratory, that was the testing ground. Once I got good at listening in my marriage, without an agenda, it overflowed to my friends and family, and then I was ready to bring it into the treatment room with my patients.

*

Here is Arjuna. He will share with you a couple of nuances that he shared with me in our coaching, and that we can use to deepen our ability to listen.

Active Listening

Active listening means that you use your language to affirm that you have fully heard what the patient has shared with you. It doesn't mean mimicking or parroting exactly what they said word for word, which would sound strange. We do use language to make it clear that the patient has been heard, that we empathize and understand.

For example, your patient might say, "I have noticed a lump under my right armpit. It has been there for several weeks, and at first I thought it was just a swollen lymph node. But I started to look online, and I asked my friend who is very intuitive, and now I feel very worried. I don't want to jump to any hasty conclusions here, but something feels very off."

Active listening would allow you to say, "Yes, I hear that you feel concerned. Initially you thought that it was nothing, but now that it has been a few weeks and you have some other input, you want to know what is going on."

As you can see, you are not adding anything new to what your patient said, you are simply adding reassurance, in your own words, that you have heard what was said.

If you were to say, "Well, your intuitive friend may not be qualified to offer an opinion," or "Don't worry, it's probably nothing," or "You should have come in sooner," you have shifted from active listening to offering your own opinion.

Deep Listening

Deep listening means not only hearing the content of what your patient says and fitting it into what you think you understand, but also sensitively paying attention to the emotion with which they say it, and their body language. It also means paying attention to the emotions that are implied, but not fully owned or expressed. It means paying attention to the obvious things that someone might feel in that situation, and giving that space. It means paying attention not only to what is said with words, but also to what has not been said, but is implied. Deep listening means listening with all of you, not just with the mind.

This takes a little time for it to become natural and graceful, but here are a few ideas to get started with:

If you feel a strong emotion in your own body, that you suspect may be more to do with your patient than with you, you might ask, "Hmm. Do you feel sad/angry/frustrated... about this?"

If your patient puts a lot of energy into defending a position, ask gentle questions to see if they are also avoiding the opposite. For example, if your patient says, "I absolutely know that this condition has nothing to do with emotions or stress, it is purely physical," you might ask, "I see. And if there was any emotion involved, what would it be?"

If your patient refers to a feeling or belief that seems unreasonable or forbidden to feel, you can create a safe container to express it. "Many people might feel angry in a situation like this..."

You can also use stories from your professional experience, or even from your own life. "I know that when I also have had similar symptoms, I felt afraid and powerless. It's natural to feel that way."

When learning to listen deeply, it is important that we do it for real, and that we don't simply learn how to mimic the appearance of it. It is possible to fake deep listening, even when we are not fully present to receive what is being said. Then it is just like a false smile or a mask. Deep listening is not a communication skill that you can learn, and then rehearse, and then reproduce like an actor, but is connected to whether you really care to know. It means to deeply open your heart, and to listen from your heart, with real living compassion. It comes from truly wanting to understand the other being.

Chapter Five
You are Treating People, Not Conditions

Dear Hannah,

While you were in medical school, you spent the first two years studying the healthy human body and basic sciences: physics, chemistry, biology, and then anatomy, histology, physiology. These are all ways of understanding the way that the body should function in the absence of pathology. You then spent another three years studying all the things that can go wrong, and what to do about them, including pathology, pathophysiology, pharmacology, the clinical textbooks of diseases, treatments, and surgical approaches. In the years ahead, the next challenge is to be able to make accurate diagnoses, to give the condition a name, and to follow the right course of treatment.

But this kind of diagnosis is only a small part of what really helps people to become well. Because the focus is really quite narrow: on the presenting complaint, it is only the first step. When you first meet a patient, you may ask, "Why are you here?" They will tell you a story, and you have learned to scan that story for the presenting complaint. Once you recognize the presenting complaint, you will arrive at your differential diagnosis, and you will start to think about additional diagnostics and potential treatment plans. By being trained in pathophysiology, you have learned to study an isolated set of signs and symptoms, what might cause them, what effect they might have, and which chemicals or techniques to apply to make those symptoms go away. By focusing only on the presenting complaint, we are not necessarily also paying attention to the multidimensional components of health — what constitutes a healthy human being.

The study of symptoms and how to alleviate them is extremely important for you as a doctor, and it will keep you very busy over the next six years. It is not an easy skill to learn or to master. But I also want to plant a seed in your heart: that by pursuing this too exclusively, you limit your patient to their complaints.

You limit your experience of your patients to what they are suffering from, and that does not necessarily help them, in the long run. It does not necessarily empower people on their road to real health. It may help you, as a doctor, to alleviate the problem, but if you stick only with that, you may lose sight of the human being you are dealing with.

We have not been trained to understand the anatomy of a multidimensional healthy human being, in all the different aspects of the ecosystem that makes each of us healthy. This includes what makes someone feel motivated, how they feel respected, how they feel cared for, how they feel energized, when they feel safe, and, indeed, all of the different feelings they have. Do your patients feel loved? Do they have an opportunity to fully express their love to others? Do they feel a sense of purpose?

After all the studies that you have been through, you have been given the grace to work with real people. I want to remind you that you have primarily been reading books for the last six years. You saw a few patients, here and there, but you were primarily acquiring knowledge.

You will have real patients around you now, and you will see that the determinants of their health are not as cut and dried as the ones that you have learned. Real people experience health, not only from the anatomy or physiology point of view that you have studied. They experience health determined by their sense of well-being: feeling good, feeling energized, feeling socially connected, feeling loved, feeling appreciated, feeling capable to do the things they want to do. These are some of the things that matter to people.

For example, in your anatomy class, you learned all we know about how the movement of the arm works. You learned about what the arm muscles look like, you dissected them, you learned about the bones and ligaments, and you learned about the nervous system that sends electrical impulses from the nerve endings to the brain, and from the brain to the muscles, to create movement. You learned how any of that can malfunction, and what to do to remedy it. On the other hand, the patient is more concerned to ask, "How does my arm feel?" and "Am I able to do with my arm what I want to do?" These questions are more important and relevant to them. When freedom to move in the world becomes restricted in any way, then the patient will ask themselves, "What is the impact on the rest of my life to not be able to do things with my arm?"

*

Let me tell you a story where I felt deeply reminded of all this. This story is not only significant for what happened at the time, but it's also interesting to reflect on what happened when I told the story to Arjuna, twenty years later.

I was at the hospital preparing for the night shift at 10.30 p.m. I was in the physicians' room, getting ready to receive handover. Ten patients were on intensive care, all of them critically ill. So there were many things I had to pay attention to during the night, lists of things to be done, things to be checked. Then the telephone on the desk rang. It was the helicopter emergency service. They told me that a thirteen-year-old girl named Rebecca had been found comatose in a small village in the French part of Switzerland. They had picked her up, intubated and ventilated her, and they were bringing her to the hospital with a team of three people.

As the double doors of the intensive care unit swung open, a wave of cold air swept in with the distinct smell of kerosene and disinfectant. The rain-soaked paramedic team rattled the squeaky-wheeled stretcher along the corridor at high speed. Adrenaline surged through my tingling body as I hurried ahead in an attempt to get the earliest possible impression of what was going on.

They brought her down from the helipad to the intensive care unit on a gurney and gave us what little information they had. A small team of four people were busy establishing all the monitoring, transferring her ventilation to our machine, transferring the lines, and running all the medication she was on for transport. We examined her head to toe. Her heart and respiration were stable but she was unresponsive, so we did everything we could to try to determine the possible cause of her condition. We went through all the tests, from every opening in the body. Where there was not already an opening, we made one: central venous access, blood tests, urine catheter, spinal tap, cerebrospinal fluid, you name it, there was a tube connected. We could not find anything wrong.

The family was not there yet; they were coming in their private car and would arrive later. So we decided to take her off the heavy sedation, to at least take that pressure off her body. We thought she might wake and be able to breathe on her own. Later, she was stable with adequate reflexes and we took off the ventilator.

When the parents came, they were absolutely desperate. They were in great fear about their child, and were on the phone continuously with their friends trying to figure out what could have happened, and to get information. But there was absolutely nothing. I talked to them, but all they could offer me was that Rebecca had been a little more closed down in the last days. They had not given it much attention. There was no boyfriend, no love affair, no major life event.

We tried to console her parents, and to reassure them that she was doing very well under the circumstances, and she would likely go comfortably through the night. We would just need to continue our work, and figure out what was wrong. We arranged for the parents to sleep at the hospital, and so they went to their room.

A little while later, everybody was gone. The nurses were attending to other patients, the emergency anesthetist left. Only one nurse and I were left in the room with Rebecca, but then an alarm in another room went off, and the nurse left as well.

Everything was quiet. It was peaceful, late in the night. There was no running and rushing anymore. The monitors were beeping quietly and steadily, the ventilators were quietly doing their thing on the neighboring ICU beds, almost like the purring of contented kittens.

I reviewed her charts, and reflected quietly to myself about what we had done so far with Rebecca; I asked myself how we might better understand her condition. At this point, she was not on the ventilator anymore, she could breathe by herself.

Suddenly, I felt a huge wave of sadness coming over me. I had absolutely no idea where it was coming from. I reflected for a moment, but there was nothing in my own life that would explain this feeling. I was struggling to hold back the tears as I pulled up a chair and sat down next to her.

Feeling this sadness, and not knowing where it was coming from, I just reached out and held her hand, and looked into her young, innocent face. And then, knowing that she was in a coma, and that she could probably neither hear me nor understand me, I found myself whispering, "I would really like to find out what is going on with you, and how I could possibly help you."

After a pause of less than a minute, she opened her eyes, and looked directly into my eye. Then she closed her eyes again. I sat bolt upright. What was that? She had not reacted in any way to pain. She had not flinched when we put a thick needle in her arm. There had been no response at all when we put a tube of about two centimeters in diameter down her airway. She did not react as we inserted a urine catheter into her bladder. But now, as I whisper these few simple words, she opens her eyes. Was I dreaming?

I remained there for a while longer. Then she opened her eyes again, and looked into my eyes.

"Really?" she asked very clearly.

I was blown away. I could not even answer. I just looked at her, overwhelmed by the situation. Then I nodded. "Yes. Tell me how I can help."

And so Rebecca started to tell me her story. She talked for a considerable time. The essence of it was that her cousin had sexually abused her. She thought her parents would not understand, nobody would, and the only way that she could make it stop was to die and "switch everything off inside."

It was a long night. I spent many hours with her. Luckily the ward was quiet so the night allowed for that. In the morning, I canceled all the remaining tests; we only did a few essential things to make sure that we did not miss anything. Once all of this was done, she was referred to a psychiatric unit, where she worked with a psychiatrist and a psychologist as an outpatient.

You are Treating People, Not Conditions

This is only one of many, many stories that illustrate that when we focus on the presenting condition, we frequently overlook what is really going on for the patient.

But this is only part of the story. As I mentioned, I told this story to my coach, Arjuna, during an intensive retreat we did together here in Basel. We were working on the vision for Heart-Based Medicine at the time. We sat up in the attic, where I have my office. We had a whiteboard, colored pens, recording equipment, everything we could need for a day of hard-core visioning. But after a couple of hours, Arjuna stopped me.

"You know, Jan, we are remaining very heady and conceptual. It is natural, because you are trained as a doctor and an academic. I think we need a better environment to do our work today."

Arjuna suggested that we spend the day at the zoo, which is just down the road from my house. I probably told him half of the stories in this book at the zoo that day. One case study I shared with him while looking at the elephants. Another case study was delivered to Arjuna, and also to the lions. I told this story of Rebecca to Arjuna in the penguin enclosure.

When we got to this point in the story, I told Arjuna that I referred Rebecca to the psychiatric unit as an outpatient. He asked me, "So what happened next? What happened to her? What happened to the cousin who had abused her?"

I had to tell him that I didn't know. In the medical system as it is today, all over the world, when you refer a patient to another department, you rarely hear about them again.

He paused to reflect. He looked at the penguins for a few moments. "I am curious," he said, then asked me, "Did you feel interested to find out what happened to her, and what happened to the cousin who was abusing her?"

"As a doctor, I see about thirty or forty people a day," I educated him. "It is impossible to follow up all of them."

"I understand," he said. "But I am wondering. This is such a strong moment that you shared. You felt this sadness, you held her hand, and you felt this bond. You told her that you really wanted to help her, and she opened her eyes, and said, 'Really? Do you really want to help me?' Didn't this feel a little different? Like you had a real human connection?"

I had to admit that I didn't follow up. Not only that, it also felt quite normal and routine to me that it was this way.

"Could you, if you had wanted to, could you have found out what happened to her?" Arjuna asked me.

"Yes, very easily. I could have found out."

"So why didn't you?"

"I was overwhelmed, by the next batch of patients, by their needs and requirements."

"Hmmm. How did that feel then? How does it feel now, looking back on it, to have this depth of bond with somebody, and then to never find out what happens next?"

I had to stop and think. I also looked at the penguins. They looked back at me, and waddled away. They were clearly going to offer no help. "It leaves a scar," I said finally. I was surprised to hear my voice say those words, but it was true. "It leaves a scar that does not heal."

This was a pivotal moment for me, Hannah, in the development of Heart-Based Medicine. It seemed completely normal and acceptable to me, but for

Arjuna it was difficult to understand, and he was curious to know more. He told me that he had very little reference for something like this in his life: to have this kind of depth of connection with another human being, and then just to move on to the next thing. It shed a light on so many things that have become out of balance in modern healthcare.

We treat conditions; we have forgotten the connection with people. As soon as we successfully find the correct diagnosis, the job is done, and we move on to the next bed. I realize that my medical training has made me skilled at recognizing and alleviating specific pathologies, but at the same time it has, slowly and gradually, caused a kind of blunting of my basic humanity.

This was a moment where I entered into a deep and tender trust with another human being, but by virtue of the context in which I was operating, she became just another object on the conveyor belt, another medical conundrum to solve, one which was in and out in a day. I got used to seeing myself as a cogwheel in a big system, passing the problem on to the appropriate part of the system. She was a cog in a machine, I was a cog in the machine, and temporarily we had a professional interaction until I allowed myself to feel the resonance with her and this changed her course toward healing — and also mine.

*

As you move through your training in the hospital, my hope is that you can remember that each new interaction is not just a high-blood-pressure case, or a fatty liver, or a clogged artery. Each new interaction is a living human being, with hopes and regrets, with strengths and weaknesses, with pride and with shame. Each new human being is somebody's daughter, or somebody's wife. It is someone who had a childhood, with gifts for their birthday. It is somebody who has a job, which they would like to be meaningful. This is somebody who worries about income tax. This is somebody who takes pride in their flower arrangements. This is somebody who cries when you hold their hand in the right way. And all of these very different things, or the lack of them, contribute to their overall sense of well-being.

You are dealing with this entire complex web of factors that make up human life. Any time that you try to isolate a symptom from the rest of those factors, and just aim to make the symptoms go away with a drug treatment, you have reduced yourself to a technician, rather than someone truly contributing to healing.

Please allow yourself to do exactly what you have not been encouraged to do by the medical system: take an interest in people in a multidimensional way. It does not take very long to ask people questions that bring forth their pleasures and their worries. "Oh, you are married. How is everything at home? Do you have children? How are your children doing? Do you love your work?" Simple questions like these will allow you to enter into the incredibly rich, multidimensional, complex world of unique human life. It is within that very rich and complex tapestry that you may discover the secret of their overall health, or lack of health.

*

Here are three tips that Arjuna and I have developed for you, that can help you pay more attention to the whole human being, and not get lost in focusing only on the presenting complaint and the list of diagnoses they accumulated during their patient career.

The First Five Seconds

Take note of the first five seconds in which you meet a new patient. Really feel deeply what you experience in those first moments. There is so much to learn. For example, there are some patients who uplift you, and you feel alive and light, and smiling. There are some patients where you have a hard time even breathing, and you feel pressure, weight, and suffocation.

There are all sorts of feelings, and sometimes images, that arise in the first few seconds of meeting a patient. Make a point not to race toward the diagnosis, but stop and linger for a moment on what happens in your own body, inside yourself, in those first few seconds. If you can, make a practice to jot down a few notes.

In medical school, they teach you that the first thing is to write down the presenting complaint. I would like you to add one line above that one. Write the words: "My first impression." What did I feel, what did I see, what did I smell?

Ask Irrelevant Questions

As you listen to the patient history, and you are scanning for signs and symptoms and pattern recognition, you ask questions that guide your differential diagnosis. By the time you are done with this, and you have taken your full history, make a point to also ask a few questions that are seemingly irrelevant, that are seemingly not guiding your differential diagnosis.

When you go through the personal history, expand a little beyond what seems immediately relevant, and find out what your patient likes in life, what they enjoy, what they are knowledgeable about, what drives them. This has two really important effects. First, it will loosen up the professional rigor you have been trained in, and this will help you to connect with your patients in a deeper way. But also it will allow you clues and insights into the multidimensionality of their lives, help you to understand all of the factors that effect health and sickness. When you prompt patients to talk in a more general and relaxed way, they will tell you things that end up being highly relevant to their diagnosis, things that you might not have dreamed of asking, if you had been more linear in your questioning.

What Do You Need?

The most essential question to ask your patient, as you are collecting data and getting to know them better, is "What do you need?" This means, what do you wish for? What is the outcome you want? What would be most helpful and supportive to you? If you dare to dream beyond what you think is possible or impossible, then what would you most like to create here? Asking these kinds of questions will allow you to synchronize the way you have been trained, your own intuition, and the deepest longing and values of your patient.

Chapter Six
Taking Care of Yourself is Fundamental

Dear Hannah,

You are such a beautiful young woman, so full of energy and joy and vitality, life is exploding through you. I deeply hope that you can maintain this, treasure it, and even amplify it as you continue your work as a doctor.

Your parents took great care of your health, and you have done the same as a young adult. This may not always be obvious to you; it may just seem normal. Your natural life force has a powerful effect on your patients, even though you may not be reminded of this very often in medical school or in the hospital. It makes a huge difference: whether you show up with the patient as a living example of good health and vitality, or as exhausted, caught up in thinking, overwhelmed, and stressed out.

Just imagine: if you are lying in a hospital bed, feeling weak and insecure, and having doubts about your health and suffering. You are seeking out good medical attention. How would it feel, if you suspect that the doctor might be suffering more than you are?

Being an example of health as well as a knowledgeable health expert is incredibly important, but we all forget this. When it was stressful during your studies, you would call me from time to time. We both know how easy it is to forget to take care of yourself when you feel the need to achieve a goal, or to struggle through challenges. At those times, the thing that we are striving for becomes the center of our attention, and we forget all about the one who is striving.

As you know, when you get very focused on achieving outcomes, the sympathetic nervous system becomes dominant, and the parasympathetic nervous system becomes less dominant. In such a situation, heart-based intelligence is the first thing to get thrown overboard.

As you start your residency in the hospital, you will be faced every day with an interesting paradox: a contradiction of values that is staring you in the face every time you walk through the doors and put on your white coat. You are entering into a world that is all about alleviating disease, bringing physical bodies back into health. And yet almost every day you will be asked to do things that are stressful, or detrimental to your own physical body. This is definitely better today than it was when I was a resident, but the conflict of values still remains in the medical world.

When I was a resident, I was frequently asked to skimp on my sleep. At one point I remember that I did not sleep for five days in a row. I stayed awake on black coffee, and sometimes even administered saline infusions to myself, just to stay conscious. Much of what happened for me in my residency was training in how to *not* take care of a physical body, although the job I was being trained for was how to alleviate disease. The people who were educating me about disease were impressively knowledgeable, but not particularly inspiring role models of how to take care of a human body, or to create extraordinary health. Some were smoking cigarettes, abusing alcohol, not exercising, snacking fast food, among many other habits that are not famous for creating good health.

The hospital environment often thrives on a sense of emergency. There are lives to be saved, constant fires to be extinguished. It is often viewed as selfish, therefore, or as an abandonment of responsibility, if you want to do something to take care of yourself. Hannah, I want to encourage you to understand that looking after your own body is not selfish: it is the most immediate thing you can do as a foundation for taking care of other people.

Human bodies are made out of the earth: they are like animated earth. They get all their nourishment and fuel from sunlight and plants, and everything they excrete goes back into the earth. The most immediate connection you have to this world of physicality, the arena in which you have the most responsibility and opportunity to make an immediate improvement, is in the relationship to your own body. Your relationship to all other bodies will be a direct reflection of that.

I can imagine that someday you will have children of your own. Then it will be absolutely obvious to you that the better you take care of your own body during pregnancy, the healthier those children will be. In just the same way, when you go to the hospital inhabiting a very healthy body, you have cultivated a disposition for treating other bodies with equal care and respect. You start where you have the most responsibility and opportunity to effect change: with your own body; then it extends to your children, and then it overflows into the hospital room. It is very simple. If someone

cannot give loving attention to their own body —
giving it enough sleep, good quality nutrition,
moments of rest and care, as well as moments of joy,
happiness, and loving connection — how can it be
possible to convey this feeling to others? When you are
taking good care of yourself, in every way, it will be an
inspiration to your patients. Look at your friends and
your colleagues: it is very obvious who is exuding
extra life force, happiness, and well-being, and who is
stressed out and simply performing and trying to get
through another day.

As I have said, there are many ways medical school
encourages you to ignore the needs of your own body:
encouragement to get by without sleep, to skip proper
food breaks, or to simply subsist on black coffee and
candy bars. Because of a lack of education in this area,
it creates a dominant culture. You may be around other
medical students and residents who are not taking
good care of their physical well-being. Because it is the
culture, it just goes unquestioned.

I have gone through many periods of my life,
particularly during residency, when I completely
forgot to take care of myself. It has never worked out
well. Can you imagine, I was even smoking in my
doctor's office in some of the hospitals? It was
considered normal and went unquestioned. Although I

stopped smoking long ago, smoking is prohibited on most hospital grounds and things are much better in and around the hospital today than they were for me. I teach medicine today, and I cannot really see that the general culture has shifted that much.

When you overlook the needs of your own body, there are two immediate consequences. First, you become desensitized to well-being, and you even forget what it is like to have that "yummy feeling" of pleasure in your belly for no reason. Second, once you have forgotten the feeling of extraordinary good health for yourself, you quickly lose sight of it as a possibility for your patients. Then the patients simply become functional problems to fix, instead of whole human beings who deserve to feel good. Your patient becomes "the liver in bed five," instead of Mme. Laurent, who has two daughters and five grandchildren, and who loves Mozart, loves to read a book on the back porch in the evening, with an Aperol Spritzer, who loves her family so much, but finds she has less to give to them when she feels unwell. Well-being is not simply the absence of disease symptoms: it means living within a body that is capable of joy and love for no reason.

I have had many wake-up calls in my life about taking good care of my body. One of them came at just the same stage that you are: in residency. The other one came more recently, as part of my experience of coaching.

*

At the beginning of my residency, I found a very economical place to live. It was a room in a basement, behind the garage, about three meters square, with a tiny window. I rented it from a nice couple. The benefit was that it was very cheap. In order to get to my room to sleep, I had to walk through the garage, which smelled of the car engine. In my room I simply had a small bed, and my medical books. When I wanted to wash, I used a hose coming out of the wall in the same room where the family had their washing machine, surrounded by all the clothes hanging to dry. This situation served me quite well for a while, but there was a little voice inside, reminding me that this was not really a healthy place to live. It was okay, just to have a place to sleep. But that was all.

I had grown up in a rural area near Munich, in Germany. I know what healthy food tastes like. At that time, there were almost no health food shops; they didn't exist. By chance, one of the first ones in Switzerland was near where I was living. They had a small variety of organic produce. The vegetables were three or four times the cost of what I could buy in the supermarket. A liter of cow's milk was five dollars, instead of one dollar at the supermarket. The money I was saving on rent I was spending on trying to keep my body healthy.

Then I moved to a farmhouse in Alsace, in France. It was a typical Alsatian farmhouse built with wooden beams, and the space between the beams was filled with clay and straw. In English, they call this timber framing, or "post and beam" construction. The building where I lived was two stories, with a very high roof. About one third of it was for me, up a very steep old staircase to the first floor. Everything was heated by a wood-burning stove.

This was about a 30-minute drive from the hospital, in my old VW hippie van, so it added one hour of driving time to every day. At the beginning, I was concerned. But then I really came to appreciate this time. There really was no way to make it efficient. I couldn't get anything done. So it became my time to settle … that is, whenever I was not busy keeping the parts of the van together while driving. I would go from a full day of stuffing my brain in the University library, and then have this decompression time before I returned home, where I could connect again with nature, let the mud settle in my brain, and allow a feeling of deep rest to come over my body.

I would leave the city somewhere between six and eight in the evening. Once I got home, I was already feeling more relaxed, and looking forward to this magical environment. Toward the end of the drive, as I drove into the farm, the wheels of my van were going through cow dung. I would pull into the driveway, and park in front of the barn. In the lower floor of the barn were farming machines: tractors and a plough. Upstairs was a huge loft, filled with hay. When we had a party on the weekend, this is where all my friends would sleep.

I used to come home, step out of my van, and my foot would come down on the earth. There was a meadow right next to me. Outside my front door was a little pergola, with a vine full of grapes. Everything smelled deeply of the countryside. In the evening there was moisture in the air, you could smell the warmth of the soil, you could smell the heat reflecting off the stones carrying the scents of herbs and flowers. Each season would smell different. Sometimes it smelled richly of flowers; in the autumn there was the smell of the wine and the grapes hanging in thick bunches; in the winter it smelled of rich, damp nourishment. Sometimes the entire village smelled of cut grass. After a big rain, you would smell mushroomy, mossy smells from the woods. It was always different, it was always alive. Every time I came home, there was a new surprise, and I used to look forward to asking "What does nature have in store for me today?"

The farmhouse had a long overhanging roof. I had a huge sofa there, next to the front door. I used to throw my bag down on the sofa, go inside, and bring out something to drink and a snack to eat. I was growing my own vegetables already, so instead of going shopping, I would walk into the backyard to see what was ready. Sometimes there was a nice lettuce or some zucchinis ready to be plucked. Sometimes the snails got there first. I would go with whatever the garden had to offer, and then stroll back into the kitchen to prepare it. There was a butcher in the next village, and sometimes I would drive there to buy freshly killed meat, and eat it with vegetables from the garden. I used to drink tea in the evening, made from herbs that grew outside my window. Sometimes I could afford a bottle of wine, which also came from a local vineyard.

Naturally, I went to bed earlier. When I lived in the city, it was always after midnight, and sometimes as late as 2 a.m. Now, living in the countryside I was in bed before 11. I had the windows open at night, so I could fall asleep with the fresh air. At night it was completely quiet, and totally dark. The crowing of the cock and the church bells were my alarm clock.

This life created an incredibly important separation between the hectic pace of the hospital and my downtime. The drive made it very clear that outside of the city is not for work, and inside the city is where work happens. Of course, I did write my thesis in the farmhouse, but it was a completely different environment. It felt more like a place to be creative than to have to apply any pressure. Do you remember, I wrote you in a previous letter about the two wolves? Both wolves benefited from this lifestyle. I became more efficient during the day, I had more to give at the hospital, and I learned everything more quickly when this nurturing wolf also had an environment and time for me to take care of myself.

Your father, Dominik, used to visit me all the time. He was my best friend. He used to love coming to the farmhouse. We had both grown up in the countryside, each in a small village. He had a flat in Freiburg at the time, so it was not very far to travel. He used to call my place his "country house." We used to go for walks together.

At that time, Dominik was doing a thesis that involved experiments with chickens. He was using a gene gun, loaded with tiny gold particles, and shooting them into the ovaries of chickens, to see if instead of producing ovalbumin, they could produce another protein to be used as drugs or vaccines. He was getting fertilized eggs every day from a local farmer so he could catch the chickens, and then, when they were just the right size, he would use his gene gun.

Around this time we had a discussion, sitting on my outdoor sofa together one evening. We decided that we should really not be eating meat, unless we were actually able to raise the animals ourselves. It felt like a kind of cheating. We made a pact together, like brothers, that either we would both quit eating meat altogether, or we were going to raise and kill the animals we ate.

One day he came with six eggs and a warming lamp that people use for hatching. It was actually my birthday. He came with an architect friend of his, who had an elaborate plan for a very impressive henhouse, with a drawbridge and all of the finest features. Dominik and his friend went roaming around the nearby farms asking, "Do you have a hammer... do you have a few nails... do you have a few pieces of wood lying around?" Like this they built the henhouse. They put a strong fence all around it, because there were foxes in the area.

Once the eggs were hatched, I fed the chicks scraps from the vegetables I was growing in the garden. I also went to one of the neighboring farmers who had fresh corn, and I bought a 100 kg bag to feed the chickens. Like this, we had six chickens who became very fit and healthy. We had a great time together; they became like family. I gave each chicken a name.

Finally, the day came when your father came over and said, "Jan, I think it's time to kill the first of our chickens." We had no experience. We had never killed a chicken before; in fact, we had never killed anything. We went to the neighboring farmer, and he gave us a step-by-step guide on how to kill a chicken with a machete knife. He also told us that as soon as the chicken was dead, you must immediately put it in a pot of boiling water, so the feathers come off. On the way home, we stopped at the bar and drank several rounds of whiskey: it felt like an essential prerequisite for the task ahead.

First we had to catch the chicken. If you have never caught a chicken, it is not a straightforward thing to do. We spent a good part of an hour chasing the chicken we had chosen. It was flapping its wings, scratching its claws, and pecking with its beak. I think this chicken had a pretty good idea that our intentions were not friendly. She was fast, she was fierce, but finally Dominik managed to grab the chicken, put the head down on a piece of wood, and I cut it off with the machete. I had developed a very close personal relationship with this chicken; I had been talking lovingly to her every morning. The whole enterprise was extremely difficult for me. Blood was squirting everywhere, while the body was still completely active, even without the head. We were covered in blood: clearly not professionals. We had prepared the pot of boiling water, we put in the chicken, and sure enough the feathers came off very easily.

Because Dominik was in training as a surgeon, we agreed that he was the best candidate to take the chicken apart, but then it was my job to cook her. He performed chicken surgery, and then I created chicken cuisine.

"We are in France," I thought to myself. "I have all these beautiful herbs in my garden, so we are going to have Poulet a l'Estragon." I prepared it very well, having cooked this dish many times before. I used some good wine, some tarragon from the garden, and a very good sauce with fresh cream. Usually, this dish is delicious.

Finally, your father and I sat down at the table, facing each other, to eat the chicken. It felt like a very crucial moment, both in our friendship, as well as for the chicken. This was a "brothers in arms" kind of bonding moment. Right, from now on, if we want to eat meat, we need to be able to breed it, kill it, cook it, eat it, and then learn to feel good about the whole process. It has to feel right. Otherwise, we agreed we would give up eating meat, and become vegetarians.

We looked into each other's eyes, your father and me, and we declared together, "Okay. Are we going to do this now? Shall we eat the first animal that we killed ourselves?" We each raised our knife and our fork, to take the first bite.

It was disgusting.

It was an utter disaster. It was like eating a piece of leather, or the cooked sole from your shoe. We were absolutely devastated. How was this possible? We raised the chicken, we killed the chicken, we cooked the chicken. And now, when we tried to eat the chicken, it was terrible. What did we do wrong? Did we chase the chicken too long? Did we feed it incorrectly?

Here we were, two idealistic heroes, turned into two fools. These two fools traipsed back to the neighboring farmer. We explained the problem. We went through the whole story, step-by-step, and explained to him exactly how we chased it, and killed it, and how we had used the hot water to take off the wings, and then how we had cooked it. "That all sounds just fine to me," the farmer said. "But you know, I never cook anything myself. My wife does that. Let me get her."

The farmer's wife came out to greet us. We told her the whole story again. She agreed that it sounded like a delicious recipe. She just could not figure out what we had done wrong. Finally, she asked us, "How long did you cook the chicken?" I told her that it was just the normal time, about 30 minutes. She cracked up laughing. "This is not the usual kind of chicken you buy in a shop, a chicken who has been living its whole life in a cage, and not moving. Your chicken was fed on biological grain, good food, your chicken was running around, staying fit, with strong muscles. You need to cook the chicken for at least one and a half hours."

We went back, and we cooked our chicken for a much longer time. Then it tasted pretty good. We agreed that it feels much more honest and truthful and sincere to raise the meat you plan to eat, and to kill it yourself, than just to buy a slab of meat from a shelf, wrapped in plastic. Since that time, as you probably know, your father and I do not kill our own meat, but we are very, very careful of where the meat has been sourced, and we try to find local farmers who have killed the meat themselves.

I lived like this on the farm for more than two years. Finally I had to return to the city, because it was coming close to exam time, and the son of the owner where I was living needed the apartment back. But this period was an important reference point for the rest of my life. It allowed me to learn how much our external life and work, and particularly the life of the doctor, is nourished and given freshness and aliveness by having an environment where you are really taking care of yourself.

When I started the coaching relationship with Arjuna, once again I was in a phase of not taking very good care of myself. I was very busy with the vaccine-safety initiative, and working at the hospital, and having three young children. I was back into the habit of not getting enough sleep, and just throwing back a coffee in the morning before running to work. This was one of the benefits of working with a coach, that together we could remember all the habits that have served me in my life to take good care of myself. We settled on a rhythm of good self-care, which Arjuna held me accountable for.

Once again, I'm going to pass you over to Arjuna now, and he will tell you a little bit of what he knows, as a coach, about this kind of good relationship to the body.

*

Hi, Hannah! Everything Jan just told you, I also hear from almost everyone I work with. It is not only in the medical world, but equally in technology, in political leadership, among entrepreneurs... in fact, everywhere. Even people like me, who write books and coach others on how to maintain balance in life, get pulled into the story of "I don't have enough time to take care of myself in the way I would like to."

Because of the kind of society in which we live, this issue needs to be addressed in each and every coaching relationship. Most people have plenty enough business strategies, and training, and professional tips and tools, but few people really understand the mechanics of cultivating presence by taking good care of ourselves.

Taking Care of Yourself is Fundamental

Here are the most important **self-care tips** that I know of, which are easy to integrate into your life, and make the most difference.

1. **Do nothing.** Take 20 minutes or more each morning to sit silently, doing absolutely nothing. We will talk about this more in the letter that Jan has written for you called "connect with the infinite."

2. **Reconnect with your values.** This is a great thing to do after #1 above. Take a few minutes to remember why you chose to be a doctor. Jan talked about this already in his letter called "remember your initial motivation." Dedicate yourself fresh each day in alignment with these values.

3. **Move your energy.** Make sure that you take some time each day, if possible in the morning, to stretch your body, and to wake up your muscles.

4. **Supplementation.** Make sure that you are getting all the essential nutrients to feed your body and your brain. If the diet provided for you at the hospital cafeteria is not sufficient, consider bringing in your own food, or explore nutritional supplements that can keep you in peak nutrition, physically, mentally, and emotionally.

5. **Sleep.** Make sure you get enough sleep for your body type, and aim to get as much of it as possible earlier in the night (before midnight).

6. **Intentions.** Set clear intentions for each day, and create a way to make sure they happen. This will keep your daily actions in alignment with your long-term vision.

7. **Take Breaks.** Whenever you get an opportunity for a break, use it for as deep a period of rest and recreation as possible. Consider naps or staring at trees as more valuable than time on the smartphone.

8. **Take some time at the end of every day to learn from mistakes.** You'll find more about this in Jan's letter called "end of the day practice."

9. **Choose your friends carefully.** It becomes immensely easier to take good care of yourself if you surround yourself with other people who are making the same choices.

10. **Love.** Make sure that you remember to set aside a part of every day, and a part of every week which is exclusively devoted to expressing love, and to being loved. Don't just wait for this to happen as an accident, set strong intentions around it. This is about caring

attention for others, so they feel loved — not a tingly feeling of falling in love.

Chapter Seven
Trust Resonance

Dear Hannah,

I have known you since the day you were born. When you were still very little, just three or four years old, I came over to visit your father, Dominik. You were all living in Freiburg at the time. We were sitting in the garden together, each on their own chair, around a round white table. You were holding Magda, your favorite doll. Just at that moment, a car drove up. It was Jana, your best friend, being dropped off by one of her parents. When the car door opened, you jumped up, placed Magda on the chair where you had been sitting, and ran to the car, bubbling with excitement and happiness, exuding an unconditional sense of welcome.

Later, after you had been playing together for a few minutes, Jana came over to the table. She picked up Magda, to play with her. Dominik and I looked at each other, thinking that now there would be trouble. This was your favorite doll, and you were very attached to her. But you just stood to the side, looking at your friend playing with your doll, beaming from ear to ear. You were happy that she was happy. For me, this was such an unusual quality to see in a child. You were taking pleasure in her happiness, with no possessiveness.

A little later in the day, you were both running very fast across the grass, laughing loudly. Jana tripped and fell. She started to cry, her knee was grazed. As soon as she started to cry, I could immediately also see the pain in your face, although you did not cry. You were feeling her pain as if it were your own.

Just in that little play date that you had with Jana, I saw then how easily you can fall into resonance with another. You have the capacity, Hannah, to feel another's joy as your own, and to feel another's sorrow as your own as well.

I know these moments from my own life as well. I feel a kind of oneness. I feel that we are different, but also the same. In Heart-Based Medicine, we call this "resonance."

I visited your parents near Munich, soon after they got married; that was when they told me the good news that Francisca was pregnant with you. When we first spoke about it, she was still a "me." She was now a pregnant "me." She talked about the morning sickness, and the adjustments her body was going through. A few months later, the three of us sat outside together in a café in the English Garden. Your mother had started to show a little bump in her belly. By this time, she had looked at the sonograms. At this stage she was still mostly talking of herself as a pregnant "me," and very occasionally she referenced "the baby" as a third person in the family. You were still a part of her body. I also remember the day you were born. Just one day before, Francisca was pregnant Francisca, Dominik was Dominik. One day later, Francisca was not pregnant, Dominik was Dominik, and now here was Hannah. Two became three. I can remember when your mother was breast-feeding you. You looked up into her eyes, she looked back into your eyes. It seemed like you were merging in and out of being both separate and also one. Now there were two bodies, where a few days before there had been one; this allowed the feeling of oneness to remain, while there was also the perception of two.

Now that you are twenty-five years old, Francisca is in her late forties. You might still like some of the same things, and there are probably many things where you do not share the same taste, like music. You might agree on some things and you may disagree on other things. You might still have fleeting moments of feeling one, but now they will be more rare, not like when she was breast-feeding you.

These are different degrees of resonance. Low resonance means that you experience another person as completely different from you, to the point that you might feel judgmental, unsympathetic; in some cases people feel aggressive or even violent. Wars are fought in this world because different groups of people look at each other and sense "nothing like me." No sense of oneness. High resonance means that you feel another person as extremely similar to you, to the point that you might sometimes feel that the differences are only superficial, and the oneness is what matters.

I remember when I was first dating Jessica, my wife. We met at the hospital, where we were both doctors. We were both extremely busy and stressed, so we did not have much time to spare. Sometimes during breaks we used to escape to take a walk by the banks of the Rhine River in Basel. We might take a little food as a picnic, and we would chat. We were going through the process people call "getting to know each other."

"So what kind of music do you like?"

"Well, I really love Keith Jarrett."

"No way! You love Jarrett? That's crazy. I love Jarrett too. What is your favorite piece?"

"Well, the Koln Colone concert. I listen to it so often, the cassette tape is wearing thin."

"Me too!! I listen to it every few days on the stereo in my car!" It is often how couples first get to know each other. We seek out areas of mutual interest or pleasure, and it creates resonance. It creates the feeling that this person is just like me. Which are your favorite books? What kind of food do you like to eat? Who's your favorite actor or actress?

Every time we get to the point of, "Really? You love that? I love that too!" we feel a little bit more oneness, and a little bit less different. If you found yourself having exactly the same taste in absolutely everything with another person, it could get boring, and it would appear to be something like a clone of yourself. But just the right mixture of the same and different creates strong attraction between two people, and it is how couples are formed. A lot of our relationships are about finding resonance: the feeling that you are humming at the same frequency.

There are many parallels to this in the physical world. If you get a tuning fork tuned to middle C, and knock it on a hard object near to the piano, the middle C string on the piano will vibrate. The C string one octave above will also vibrate, as well as the one above that, and the one below. But the other strings will not vibrate. There are countless examples like this of physical resonance in the material world.

Whenever we experience resonance with another person, we feel more safe. We feel more understood. Something relaxes, and we feel deeply seen and at home.

Many people instinctively recognize that resonance is an intrinsic part of healing. Whenever you discharge a patient from the hospital, and send them home, you will probably tell that person, "Get plenty of rest, don't get stressed, stay home where you feel comfortable." You will make sure there is someone to take care of them. In other words, you encourage a situation of high resonance. When you feel "I have family, I have support, I'm safe," it promotes healing.

Every parent knows instinctively what to do when a child is sick: bed rest, coziness, safety, reading a book together in bed. This is a healing environment. Although we all know this instinctively, and from our personal lives, the cultivation of this kind of resonance is not emphasized in hospital training. In fact, our hospitals are often highly stressed environments; the doctor rushes in, looks quickly at the statistics, but hardly connects with the patient at all. Ironically, the way that doctors are trained in the hospital promotes low levels of resonance.

Let me tell you a story where I learned the importance of resonance in my life as a doctor.

*

As a young doctor in pediatrics, I was on one of my first hospital shifts at the accident and emergency unit. The 1860s building at the banks of the river Rhine had solid brick walls, thick doors, neon lights, and linoleum flooring. The whole place smelled of disinfectant. Pressure on the staff was high and working hours were "as needed."

There were six consulting rooms on the emergency ward. On the river side of the corridor were the surgical rooms, a resuscitation room, the nursing station, and the waiting room for children and their parents. The doctors' room was on the other side of the corridor, with three more consulting rooms, all in a row.

It was a Thursday afternoon, the day when all the private-practice pediatricians' offices were closed, so families from all over the city came to the emergency unit with their questions. Every Thursday it was jam-packed, with every one of the six treatment rooms filled all the time, and at least ten families in the waiting room.

That day, I was the doctor on call. I was very inexperienced. I needed to double check a lot and ask a lot of questions, and I wanted to take my time with each patient to make sure I did not miss anything. But they were piling up, and piling up. Every time I finished with one patient and returned to my office to complete the paperwork, I would have to walk past the waiting room, and see more and more and more people.

The nurses were doing everything they could. They were very experienced. Every time I completed one consultation and sent the family on their way, within two minutes another family had taken their place. It took me at least twenty minutes with each patient.

I realized that I would have to speed things up. I saw fathers coming out of the consulting room in the corridor, looking around impatiently. "Where is the doctor?" I saw the nurses sitting at their station, drumming their fingers. Everybody was getting nervous and discontented.

I tried everything I could think of to move a little faster. I tried speaking faster. I tried walking faster. I tried doing the examinations of the babies a bit faster. I tried writing faster. I tried to do everything faster, and consequently I began to feel very stressed.

In this state of increased tension, whenever I walked into any of the patient rooms, the baby would start to cry immediately. It might be calm before I opened the door, then, "Waaaaah."

The parents had been waiting for an hour, two hours, three hours already. They were feeling unhappy and very impatient. They had been trying to entertain their sick child, and maybe their other children who were there as well. They had been playing with the children, doing anything to soothe their pain and complaints, to distract them. Then the door opens, with some force, and in walks a young doctor with great speed. The baby starts to cry violently, and becomes completely disturbed. As you can imagine, the parents felt even more irritated.

This did not work at all well for performing the examination. It was very difficult to talk to the parents against 120dB and still get the necessary background information. They were now completely distracted by their crying child. I tried to listen to the heart and chest and to feel the tummy, but it was very difficult to hear anything when a baby is crying full-on. By speeding things up, I was actually making my own life, and the life of the parents, even more difficult. I needed to go faster, and everything took longer.

After some time, I realized that the nurses did not have this same problem. They were not so rushed. Sometimes they came into the room with me to help. Then I realized, when I went in first, the baby would start crying. When the nurse went in first, the baby would stay calm.

Susanna was a very loving, calm, and quiet nurse. Twenty-six years old, she had long blonde hair, bright blue eyes, and a slightly fuller body. She laughed almost all the time. She was a very fun-loving, heartfelt person. As she went about her duties, she would quietly sing to herself, under her breath.

When Susanna would open the door, the baby would go very quiet, and giggle. The parents would look up, very happy. It was as though sunshine was coming into the room.

After I saw this going on all day, with dozens of patients, I realized that there was a pattern, and it was something I needed to learn. Susanna always got calm, happy babies and families. I always got crying, stressed babies, and unhappy families. I needed to go fast, and it was taking a long time. Susanna had all the time in the world, and it was going more smoothly.

She was very friendly and very supportive, so toward the end of the day as things were slowing down, I asked her, "What is your secret?"

Her answer was very simple. "Doctor, the babies can feel us. If you are stressed, they can feel it. If you feel happy, they can feel it too. It's the energy." Susanna went on to tell me that she was a massage therapist, and that she was also trained in "energy healing." This made no sense to me at all at the time, but I did get a vague sense that she might know something that would lead me out of this difficult situation.

"What do you mean, the energy...?"

"Well, Doctor, try this simple thing. Just before you go into the room, pause for a few seconds. Take a deep breath, and think of someone you love. Then expand it, and feel your love for the whole universe. Then narrow it down again, and feel your love for this baby. Then open the door."

I tried it. The very next time I had to go into a room, I paused, I took a deep breath, I felt my love for my girlfriend at the time, then I expanded it to feeling love in general, and then I narrowed it down and thought lovingly about this baby. I opened the door, and voilà! No crying.

To describe this feeling of loving connection, I use the word "resonance."

Hannah, you know this from your own personal life. By now, you have had enough contact with patients to know when you feel in tune, and when you don't.

What is less apparent to most people is that we can consciously create resonance, and we know how we can do this. It is not difficult, it is something we can influence. And it does not have to be something that happens by chance. Knowing how to create this field of resonance is at the very heart of what we have been working with as Heart-Based Medicine.

As it turns out, creating this "field of resonance" is an integral part of coaching. My coach trained more than 2000 people to also be coaches, including my wife, Jessica. So he has plenty to say about this topic.

Here is Arjuna.

*

Hey, Hannah. As Jan mentioned, one way to evoke a feeling of resonance with your patient is to remember a memory of love in your own heart before you contact the patient. Our friends at HeartMath call a specific variation of this "Heart-Based Breathing." The principle is very similar to what Susanna suggested: think of someone or something you love deeply or you appreciate. Take a deep breath, and absorb that feeling deep in your heart. Then let it expand as far as you can imagine, so it becomes a universal feeling. Take another deep breath. Then, with the out breath, focus this feeling of love onto the patient you are about to connect with.

Another method which works very well is sometimes referred to as "giving and taking with the breath." It is quite simple and easy to learn. Here are the steps:

1. Bring some attention to your own internal state, just for a few moments. Notice the thoughts that are passing, the emotions you can feel, and body sensations.

2. Imagine something like a window in the middle of the chest. With your *in* breath, imagine you can draw in all of the thoughts and feelings and body sensations through the "window of the heart" and into presence, or consciousness.

3. With the *out* breath, breathe out a sigh of blessing, where you re-create thought and feeling from out of your own presence. Repeat steps two and three a few times.

4. Now, simply expand the circumference of the breathing in to include things outside yourself. This means, you can include the thoughts and feelings of your patient. Breathe everything in through the window of the heart into presence, everything you have attributed as part of "me," and everything you have thought of as part of "the other."

5. Send out a wave of blessing, from out of your own presence, blessing the thoughts and feelings you think of as "me" as well as the thoughts and feelings you think of as "the other."

*

Initially, all of this may sound a little esoteric and strange. But it has a long history. It is known as "tonglen" and it is been the central practice in Tibet, even preceeding Tibetan Buddhism.

Connie Kishbaugh was a senior research nurse at UC Davis Medical Center, in California. This was a very demanding and stressful position. She found herself caught in the middle between the demands of patients (who were often terminally ill) and the doctors (who often were rushed and stressed). She learned this simple practice of breathing in and out, of absorbing and sending blessing, and it completely changed her experience of working with patients.

Since this practice could be a little challenging to learn from a book, we have created for you an audio recording which guides you through the steps, as well as Connie's full story, in her own words. You can get both these things when you register your copy of this book at heartbasedmedicine.org/registerbook

Trust Resonance

Chapter Eight
Don't be Afraid to Break the Rules

Dear Hannah,

As you know, your father and I have been friends since we were both children. You may also know that neither of us always obeyed the rules. In fact, some of the most creative and vivid memories of my life are with your father, being rebels and breaking rules.

In the last twenty years of being a doctor, many of the moments when I consciously and deliberately chose to break the rules were among the most valuable. This may sound strange to you, because you are in a process now that is all about learning the rules. In fact, the more you stick to those rules, the better you do in medical training.

As you go through these next years, I would encourage you to do two things. First of all, remember that every rule was originally made for a good reason, so it is always helpful for you to remember why that rule was made in the first place.

Let's think of an example. Maybe several years ago a patient's relative brought some food into the hospital that did not mix well with their medications, and the patient became very sick, or even died. Many years later you learn of a rule that no one is allowed to bring in food from the outside. This rule was created to make sure that the same mistake never happens again. But now the unconditional application of this rule also means that no patient can ever benefit from good fresh home-cooked meals brought in by loving relatives. Every rule is like this. It has an intelligent beginning, but if it is applied too rigidly or universally, it can also have negative consequences.

Second, you will need to learn how to break rules sometimes with intelligence and grace. As you gain seniority and become more autonomous, you will learn that every rule is in fact more like a guideline. They are there to support you, but they are not set in stone.

There will be people who tell you that all rules are unbreakable, and such people will strictly enforce them. But I am telling you now, dear Hannah, that nothing is set in stone. Once you understand why the rule was made in the first place, then you can also understand how it can be applied intelligently. You can adhere to the rule when you can see that it applies, or you can break the rule with grace, and intelligent people will understand. I am not recommending that you go against the regime, or become a rebel without a cause, and get into endless trouble. I am suggesting that you develop a habit for self-determination, and decision-making that you can firmly stand behind.

As you gain more and more confidence and autonomy, I can tell you now that when you look into a patient's eyes, what will matter most is not whether you adhere to the rules, but whether you are being truly authentic and obeying the unwritten rules of love. You will learn the rules of the hospital, and digest them well. You can integrate them when you feel they are applicable. When a rule does not work for you, you must also know how to take a stand for intelligence and compassion. The key thing is this: when you look one of your patients in the eye, and you have to repeat to them the current rules, can you say it with authenticity and integrity, or does it require a compromise of your heart's intelligence?

Now let me tell you a story of one of the many times when I broke the rules. It was one of the most important and pivotal decisions of my career as a doctor, and one that I will always feel proud of.

*

One cold, gray February morning, I was standing in the corridor of the hospital about to do my rounds with another specialist and four residents. Just then, one resident's cell phone rang. She was already feeling a bit stressed; she put the phone down and immediately her tone became very urgent. "Dr. Bonhoeffer, we need you in room B21 downstairs — now. There is a nine-month-old baby in respiratory distress."

We rushed down the concrete emergency stairs to the floor below. The door to the room in question was already open, and the atmosphere inside was hectic. The resident ran nervously into the room ahead of me, and I walked in behind her. Three nurses were leaning over a baby cot, dressed in yellow gowns, face masks, and gloves. The monitors were beeping; they were assisting the child's respiration with oxygen, bag, and mask. This was a baby in droplet isolation — with an infectious airway disease. The baby was suffering from spinal muscular atrophy. As you know, this is a genetic disease, where a baby is born with weak muscles, and they get increasingly more floppy with time. This baby girl, named Jasmina, had such acute bronchiolitis that she had to work hard to breathe. In these kids, a simple chest infection is a common cause of death, because they don't have the muscle strength to breathe hard enough and to clear the lungs of phlegm.

The baby's mother was standing off to the side, observing the scene. She was a strong woman, with long, dark hair. She had a very loving, caring radiance. But she was very afraid at this point, very concerned and constricted; her shoulders were shrugged up to her neck. She was clearly expecting, and afraid of, the death of her child. But she was also excluded from the scene, because of all the nurses crowded around the bed. "It's fine," I thought to myself, looking at the monitor and the team. "We have some time. Let them fiddle with bag and mask, and I'm going to take care of Mommy."

"Good Morning. I am Dr. Bonhoeffer, one of the consultants here. I have gathered what is going on. We are going to take very good care of this situation. We have time. Let's walk over now and be with your baby." I put my arm around the mother's shoulder, to give her comfort. She introduced herself as Mrs. Sabine Shah.

We walked over to the cot together, and there was little Jasmina, working hard to get enough oxygen to stay alive. "Thank you so much," I said calmly to the nurses. "We are going to stop all this now. Thank you, you've done a great job. I will take it from here." I told all but one nurse that they could go to attend to the many other patients on the ward.

I took the suction tube, and went down deep into Jasmina's airways. I sucked out a good amount of mucus. I was gently moving the catheter up and down, which made her retch and bring up some more. She still had quite a strong cough impulse: exactly what I wanted to stimulate and see. Then we put her on oxygen, and let her settle down.

"Why don't you just put your hand on her head for a moment," I said to Mrs. Shah, "so she can really feel that you are there. You can't pick her up right now, because that would not work well, but you can let your baby know that you are here."

Fortunately, Jasmina settled a bit after a while and we sat down together next to the cot. "This is very intense for you, isn't it?" I said.

"Yes, it is."

Less than a year before, Sabina had given birth to Jasmina. We could both see that now the baby would not live very much longer. At the time, there was no medication available for this kind of condition, and typically babies died younger than eighteen months. I wanted to take a moment to see where Sabina was sitting, in this journey between the birth of her little baby and her death. She seemed very quiet, and to understand that her baby was going to die soon. She was simply in shock that it could suddenly be today. She told me they had another older child, who was with a family friend, Jasmina's godmother. We spent more than an hour talking. I wanted to find out what this young mother really wanted. Did she want us to do everything we could to save the baby's life, or did she want us to create a peaceful transition? After we had taken some time to weigh the options together, I left mommy and baby together, and agreed that I would be back immediately, should Jasmina's condition deteriorate. I went back to my rounds.

When I came back that afternoon to check in, we stood on each side of the cot: Sabina on one side, me on the other, with Jasmina between us.

"How can we best support you?" I gently asked Mrs. Shah.

"I don't want her to have any pain," she said. "I don't want her to feel short of breath. I don't want her to suffer more than she needs to. I know she is going to die soon."

"We don't know for sure if she will die in the hospital this time or not," I reassured her. "It may be that she lives a few more years, it may be that she dies tonight, we cannot tell. It is best for us to follow her. She will let us know, if it is her time or not. But I do need to know what is most important to you? Do you want her to stay alive at any cost? Do you want us to use intensive care treatment? Ventilation?" I listed many other interventions. "If you don't want all of that, please tell me the things that you want to make sure absolutely do happen."

Suddenly, Mrs. Shah became very quiet. She looked right into me. "I want her to feel our love. That's all I want. That is the key thing."

"How can we support you in that?" I asked. "What should this look like?"

She did not hesitate for a second. "I would love to see her taken out of this baby cot. I would love to have a real bed, where we can both sleep together, rather than sleeping on this little bench on the side of the room. I would love for my husband to also be here, so Jasmina could lie between us."

"You know," I replied, "this is totally against hospital policy. It would mean breaking the rules. But we are going to do exactly what you say, because I can see that it is the right thing."

And that was what happened. I asked the nurses to bring two adult beds into the room.

"But... the rules... but... the acquisition forms," they each replied. "But... the administrator... but... the maintenance department... but... my job is at stake..."

"Please, just do it. I will take full responsibility. Please bring in two adult beds, and remove the cot. We are going to do this now." This decision happened at exactly three o'clock in the afternoon, when luckily there was a shift change. It was easier to get it all done because one group of nurses was going home anyway, and another group was just arriving. Each group felt the weight was carried by more shoulders.

The nurse who came on duty was one of my favorites, with a very "big mama" energy. She understood immediately. She helped the family to create exactly the setting they wanted. The two beds were pushed together. We changed the lighting: switched off the fluorescents, and we brought in soft lamps. Sabina gave us her silk shawl to hang over the lamp, we had a real candle in the room, and we collected together many other beautiful things typically not allowed in a hospital.

When Jasmina's father arrived, he was astounded. "What is going on here?" he asked.

"We are creating a space for you and your wife and Jasmina, so you can all be together for the night, and you can all be comfortable."

Their baby was deteriorating seriously. I was careful to instruct the nurses that the family does not want to go to the intensive care unit, and we had got the necessary clearance. We gave her some medication to calm her, and then they all three lay in the bed together. In the early evening, I called Jessica, my wife. "Sweetheart, I cannot come home for dinner tonight. I need to be here. I cannot leave." Luckily, as a doctor she did not need any explanation. She could immediately feel what was going on.

Finally, very late in the evening, I prepared to go home. "I am going to leave you now," I said to the family, "to go home for a little rest. Here is my cell phone number." This was also totally against the rules. You are not supposed to give your private cell number to a patient, but I did it anyway, because it was the right thing to do. I passed the case over to another doctor who was there for the night shift. She was a young colleague, with little experience of handling such situations.

At two o'clock in the morning, I got a call on my cell. It was Mrs. Shah. "This is totally not working," she told me. "The doctor here is going frantic, she is in a panic. She keeps telling us that our baby is dying, and we need to move her into intensive care. We are totally lost here. You said I could call you. Please could you come?"

This was a very tricky situation. I was at home, not on duty, and another colleague was now in charge. But you know what, Hannah? I was willing to do whatever I had to do, so that this family could have a peaceful death for their baby. When I arrived at the hospital, I went straight to the room, and my young colleague was there. "What are you doing here, in the middle of the night?" she asked me, suspiciously. "You are not supposed to be working now."

"I got a call from the mother. She was really desperate."

"Why? Why would she call you?" she asked, tersely.

I was in a very awkward position. Sometimes when we are trying to satisfy many people at the same time, we get caught between conflicting values. In this case, I did not want to offend my colleague, and create a situation where she felt distrusted. I also did not want to betray my own integrity: it is generally very important to me to be truthful. Above all, I was fully committed by now for this baby to have a peaceful transition.

"I've known the family for a very long time," I heard myself saying, "and that is why she called me." My colleague accepted the explanation, and we got ourselves a pass. "I know you have a full emergency unit tonight. Why don't you take care of the other patients. I am happy to stay here with my friends."

I spent the rest of the night there in the room with the family. I was helping to manage the situation, just fine-tuning, so everybody could be comfortable. I worked together with the night nurse; we had a set of different medications we could use. We lowered the lights to the minimum. We created an environment where this baby could let go peacefully, even with shortness of breath, and impending respiratory failure. During those few hours when I was gone, they had done four blood tests, with needles in her finger and her heel. We did not do any more tests. Things calmed down again, and everything was quiet. Jasmina was sleeping. I talked softly with the parents.

Slowly, a sacred atmosphere came over this room. Whenever any of the nurses came in, they could feel it. It was a good place. Both the parents became very happy, and at one point we were all crying together. They knew this was goodbye, but it became the most beautiful goodbye possible. We made a clear agreement that we would use the minimum of medical interventions, we would just do what we needed to do so that Jasmina could cruise through this experience, and let go peacefully.

The whole situation was unbelievably touching. We were able to speak deeply about death. "What does it really mean to die?" we could ask.

Early in the morning, a family friend arrived who was trained in craniosacral balancing. He held Jasmina's head, very tenderly. She responded well and fell into a very deep relaxation; she was breathing more efficiently and more easily.

The next shift of nurses arrived. They were completely disoriented. "Whoa! What is happening here?" they asked. "This is different than how you have been trained," I explained to them quietly. "We are not playing by the usual rules in this situation." Somehow, they accepted; they could feel that there was value to this.

A little later that morning, Jasmina died, with her head in her mother's lap. Her father was sitting next to Sabina. Their craniosacral friend was sitting on the other side. I was sitting on the bedside, with the medication ready if it was needed. Jasmine's godmother also came.

I am sure that this is the most beautiful death for which I have ever been present. Sadly, I have witnessed many. She just let go, completely at peace. It was clear to everyone: that this was the right time. None of us were crying anymore; it became extremely still in the room. This little baby's presence completely filled the room as she left. It was very different from how these things often end up happening: in an atmosphere of emergency and fear. It was as though a light was shining brightly. Everybody stayed completely still, without speaking a single word, for more than an hour. I didn't even look at my phone. I had told the resident to manage the rest of the ward, and that I would be at available only if it was absolutely urgent.

I told the family that they could be there in the room as long as they wanted. I told the nurses that the family could be there all day, if that's what they needed. I also told them that it was not necessary to take the dead body to the mortuary immediately. Everybody could stay in this temple as long as they needed to be there.

More and more and more broken rules.

When I came back after a few hours, the parents were about to leave. "We are going now, to get something to eat, because we have not eaten for a very long time," they told me. Mrs. Shah came to me, and she hugged me. "Thank you so, so much," she whispered, choking with tears. Then Mr. Shah also approached me. He was a big man, from Persia. We embraced, and we cried together. There we were, holding each other, in the middle of the corridor, for five minutes, just standing there. This is not normal practice in a hospital. It is very unusual to find a consultant on call holding another man in the corridor for five minutes, crying together. They left, a little more composed. The next day, there was a little ceremony in the chapel, which I attended.

Mrs. Shah decided to create a foundation for families who have lost a child, or who were facing the imminent death of the child. She called it the Jasmina

Soraya Foundation. She asked me if I wanted to be on the board of their foundation, as a physician. I didn't even have to think about agreeing or not. It was clearly the right thing to do. Since then, she has done incredible work to support families in similar situations. She has a very simple grassroots approach: it spreads through word of mouth. I have told many families that this kind of support is available. I have met with Sabina many times since then, sometimes in a beautiful park, or at their home. Sometimes families invite her to the hospital, after she gets to know them, to be present at the passing of their child. I have gotten to know many families through this network, and sometimes the families invite me also to the hospital, once I have become a real family friend. Sabine is now also advising the Heart-Based Medicine Foundation.

*

Hannah, I don't know how long it may take till you find yourself in a situation like that. Maybe it will be a while, maybe never. But here are a few things you might like to take away from this story.

First thing is: you may often find that the environment where people are going through important life changes is not exactly the same as you would choose, from your own care and intelligence. Sometimes you may notice that the neon lights, the linoleum floors, the easily washable walls, the plastic trays, and the microwaved food are not right. Sometimes you may also become aware that some of these things need to change, at least temporarily, so that people can get what they really need.

For so long, I just accepted that this was the way things have to be. I have been with people in states of great vulnerability, wanting to relish their last moments with their loved ones, fully faced with their weakness and suffering. Then I can often feel that the hospital environment needs a little adjustment. It took me a long time to find the courage to do this. For many years I took it as a given, something over which I had no control. But that is not true. When you act with clarity, with calm and with love, you often have the freedom to create the environment that will support your patients.

There is another thing that can be helpful. I have already told you a little bit about the work I have done with Arjuna as my coach. One of the most transformative things he has helped me to experience is that I am not really one person, not just one Jan. We are all of us actually many different parts, each of which becomes active at different times. Sometimes I am Jan the doctor, the serious physician, sometimes I am Jan the father, very loving and playful, sometimes I am critical Jan, sometimes grumpy Jan. It is important to be aware of which part is dominant in any moment, and for any decision.

When it comes to your relationship to rules, these different parts will each behave differently. One part is something like a conformist, motivated to obey the rules, who thrives on approval from authority figures. That part of us will simply develop an obedient attitude to the rules, no matter what.

We all of us have another part which is something like a teenager. This is the rebel, who will break rules simply for the sake of being rebellious. That part of us loves to give the finger to authority. If we act from that part, it will simply create conflict, difficulty, and probably induce some kind of disciplining. There is also a part of all of us that feels confused, weak and disoriented, who perpetuates the story "There's nothing I can do, I have no power, I know better, but I cannot act."

If we take action from any of these parts, which each have their separate agenda, it usually does not work out well. As soon as we have some awareness of these parts, and we can recognize the voice of conformity, the voice of rebellion, or the voice of confusion, it is also possible to take a deep breath, and to let it all go. Then you can relax into the heart of love. You will relax into the most loving, caring things that you can do for your patients, which may sometimes align with the rules, and may sometimes require you to have the courage to break the rules, and then to stand up with dignity and to defend your decision when it is questioned. You may observe that when you break rules from this disposition, it is hardly ever questioned.

The reference point is always love. The easiest way to stay connected with love in these moments is to make decisions together with the patient and their family, not outside of the room behind the patient's back. When you are connected with a real human being, there is much more likelihood of a loving decision than if you are alone, looking into your computer screen, and going through rational arguments in your head.

There is something I have realized, late in my career, that I hope you will see more quickly than I did: every patient is different and unique. It may be that the majority of people you see are served by applying the general medical rules and medical wisdom. But then there are the outliers, people who lie at the extremes of the Gaussian bell-shaped normal distribution. If you can see each person as an individual, rather than as a statistic mean, if you use love as your reference point, you will be able to best serve the patient in front of you and to follow rules and to break rules with grace and wisdom.

Chapter Nine
Question "Normal"

Dear Hannah,

When you were only about three years old, you were very curious, very nosy, you wanted to know everything. You learned to walk early, and after that you were always running at high speed to every corner that you could possibly explore. You would open every drawer, every cupboard, everything that you could reach.

On one particular occasion, I was sitting together with your father, Dominik, in the kitchen of his apartment, talking about our medical studies. We were looking at anatomy books, having a discussion about what is a normal human body.

Question "Normal"

You were happily playing in the corner when you discovered the kitchen drawer. We were absorbed in our conversation, so not watching you closely. You pulled open the drawer, and everything fell out onto the floor, on top of you. You were crying like crazy. Dominik remained very calm and collected, he picked you up, held you quietly until you settled, and then said, "Hannah, that was not such a great idea. Let's figure out together how we can put the drawer back in shape, and put everything away again." Once again, I was very impressed with the way Dominik handled this and thought to myself, "This is how I wish to handle these situations, when I have kids."

Finally we sat down together again to talk about the "normal" human body. Dominik offered the parallel of what had just happened with the drawer. Pulling the drawer out, causing everything to fall on the floor could possibly be seen as a symptom of aberration: an unhealthy behavior that needs to be "cured." Or you could simply see it as a healthy sign of curiosity.

How do we understand what is "normal"? Often it simply means behavior that is more convenient for adults (when speaking about a child) and later it means behavior that is more easily controlled: by governments or by employers.

As you go through the next years as a young doctor, you will be invited to compare everything against Gaussian normal distributions. You know what those charts look like: almost no activity on the far left or the far right, with a big bump in the middle. You will be encouraged to steer patients back into the middle of the distribution: physically, psychologically, and behaviorally. Anything outside two standard deviations of the mean of what we have agreed is "normal" you will be encouraged to view as a pathology, something to be "healed" so that your patient conforms with our idea of how people should be. Abnormalities are often viewed as problematic.

There have been many moments in my career as a doctor where I had doubts about the way we define "normal." When I was an elective student at Oxford University in England, we had a wonderful consultant in pediatric gastroenterology. He introduced me to a book called *The Normal Child*. Sadly, that book is no longer available. Otherwise I would have sent you a copy a long time ago. The book highlights the most frequently observed characteristics of a child by age. How long does a child sleep? How often does a child pee? This book shows the variables of normal. It helped me to appreciate the huge variance, and also that a child can be way outside of the big bump in the middle of the Gaussian curve, and still be completely healthy, and beautiful. Developmental pediatrics is now the young specialty looking more deeply into this and also seeing the child with its peculiarities in its social context. I recommend you to follow the developments in the specialty closely. They are developing something fundamental for medicine in general.

Sometimes, our idea of "normal" is defined by how easily people can function in a commercial society. If you can go to work, if you can make money, if you can keep your head down and not draw attention to yourself, if you can remain satisfied with the entertainment, food, and lifestyle marketed to you, then all is well. You are "normal." If you do not fit into the cogs of organized society, you are regarded as pathological. But what if some of the assumptions we make about organized society are themselves not truly healthy? Think about the popular myth of lemmings running at high speed over the edge of a cliff to their death. If one lemming were to go against the crowd, the other lemmings might call this rebel "abnormal," or even pathological. But looked at from the outside — from an ontological perspective — that is the only healthy lemming in the social system. That is the only lemming that is not suicidal.

I have had many important moments in my career as a doctor where I was able to question "normal." Let me tell you about one of those times now.

*

I was a junior resident in the hospital. The corridor on that ward had a slight bend in it. There was a whole line of rooms on one side, and then on the other side of the bend was another set of rooms. Right in the middle, at that bend, was another corridor going in another direction, at right angles. I could stand in that place, look to my left, and see all of the patient rooms in that direction. If I turned my head to the right, I would see all of the other rooms.

One morning, I was standing in this corridor, starting to make my rounds. I had a little trolley in front of me with all of the paper records and radiographs for all of the patients. I knew this was going to be a very busy day, with eighteen children, some very sick, and some only in the hospital temporarily. At this moment, the telephone rang.

"We are going to move six patients to your ward today. By about lunchtime, please make sure you have freed up six spaces." I was already feeling a little overwhelmed, but now this gave me a lot of extra work. I was going to have to discharge six patients, to free up six rooms. I asked about the new patients coming in. Two of the children had cerebral palsy of unknown cause, another had a severe muscular disorder, another had severe epilepsy. These were not children coming in temporarily to the hospital with bronchitis or diarrhea. These were the kind of children who lived more or less permanently in a hospital.

"But don't worry," the voice on the phone said. "They all have extensive medical records. We have them here, a big thick folder for every child. We are going to send all the records down to you."

I started immediately to go on my rounds, and sure enough it was quite easy to discharge six patients that morning. I even had enough time to go to my office and to browse through these thick binders on the new children coming in. The more I read, however, the more overwhelmed I felt. I did not feel qualified to manage the complex care of these patients. None of them conformed in any possible way to our idea of "normal." I called the neurologist. "These are your patients," I said. "I am not familiar with these kinds of situations. Please, could you come over and walk me through how to manage them." He agreed to come over later in the afternoon.

The discharged children left in the morning, and by lunchtime the new children, who needed much more long-term care, had arrived. By early afternoon, everything had quietened. I had to walk back from my office through this slightly bent corridor. It so happened that these six new children were all in rooms in a row. I had to walk past their rooms before I could get to the other patients. It was the middle of the afternoon already, and the nurses had helped these new patients out of their beds, to sit in chairs on the corridor, and to enjoy the sunshine and the view. I had to literally pass by one... two... three... all six of the wheelchairs, each one with a severely disabled child: high muscle tone, very distorted bodies, dribbling saliva. Their heads were turned upwards, their eyes wandering about in a very undirected way.

I felt ashamed.

I knew that I was responsible for these children, but I also knew that I didn't have a clue. On top of this, I had no idea how to interact with them, because all of my experience was with "normal" children. If I would speak, or smile at one of these children, I got just a strange response, or an empty stare. I felt completely helpless. On the outside, I walked by and just said "Hello." But inside, I was feeling constricted.

Question "Normal"

Once I got to the other side of the ward, past the bend in the corridor, everything felt familiar again, and I felt comfortable. Here was a six-month-old baby with diarrhea, with the mother. Here was a six-year-old, with bronchiolitis, watching television. These were children with diseases, who were otherwise normal.

A group of nurses was standing there together at their station. They all turned around at the same time, and looked at me. I wondered what I had done.

"What's going on with you?" one of them asked me. They could all see I was not happy, not comfortable. They could see I was agitated. I confessed that I was feeling disturbed inside. I did not know how to handle the situation with these new children.

"Is this the first time you are seeing disabled kids?" One of the nurses smiled at me, with innocent curiosity.

"No, of course not. But this is the first time I have ever felt responsible for them. I remember, as a judo teacher, once I was teaching blind people. It was actually very rewarding, because they could feel things that I was totally unable to experience. Those blind kids taught me a lot about how much more you feel when you cannot see. They used other senses than I was using."

"So, what's the problem?" this nurse continued. Those kids before, they couldn't see. These kids today, they can't move or speak. What's the difference?"

I left the nurses' station, feeling confused. I knew that somehow I had to break through. So deliberately I went back to that same place in the corridor where it curves. I just stood there. On the right side were all the "normal" children, watching TV, talking with the parents, doing all the things I was familiar with. On the left side were the disabled children.

The child closest to me on the left side was an eight-year-old boy called Frank. He had cerebral palsy, as a result of having had measles encephalitis as a baby. His body was completely distorted. He had head support, and very heavy side supports. He was strapped into a red wheelchair with several thick seatbelts to keep him in a fixed position. He was drooling heavily, so a napkin had been placed under his chin to catch the saliva. He had a strange haircut that looked like it had been done with garden shears.

Suddenly, from out of this distorted body strapped into the wheelchair, his eyes opened large, and he was looking directly into me. His eyes looked so warm, so deep, so wide, and so unconditionally loving. I experienced tremendous light coming from this being. He became extraordinarily beautiful to me.

I stood there, and we looked into each other, transfixed, for maybe ten or fifteen minutes. I was amazed by how he could hold this gaze with total attention, given how distorted his body was. Suddenly, a huge space opened up inside of me. For a few moments, there was no Frank, there was no Dr. Bonhoeffer, there was no more two of us. All of this was gone. There was just connection.

There was just love.

Hannah, I have experienced this kind of gap in time before. Most people love small babies. When you look into the eyes of a small baby, you are drawn into an innocence and purity. Everybody longs for that. I have also had the opportunity to be close to people who have absorbed themselves in a lifetime of mystical experience and practice: people who have spent decades in meditation. I have experienced the same kind of melting and merging there too. I have also been around many people who were in the process of dying. At that time, we let go of all our attachments. There it is again, that kind of translucence. At these times, a window opens and then aaaaah..., you are connected again. You are no longer separate from the source that gives you life.

Then that window closed, and once again here was Frank, the cerebral palsy patient, and here I was, the doctor, feeling scared, standing in the corner.

In that moment I had a strange and illogical insight. From a certain perspective, this boy was more healthy than I was, and actually more healthy in some ways than the children on the other side of the ward. He had a capacity for tremendously deep connection.

I turned to look to my right. In every single room the TV was running, there was noise. People were talking, laughing. There was also connection, but it was a different kind.

After that, I had no more fear of being with these disabled patients. I could often meet them in a much more direct way than I could meet the others. It did not require any talking, it did not require me to put on any kind of act or persona. I just had to be there, and show up.

That day, a lot changed in how I perceive myself as a physician, how I meet patients, and how I define "healthy" and "unhealthy," and what is "normal" and what is "abnormal."

From a conventional medical perspective, Frank had a very complex health situation that made him very sick. Medicine today describes the characteristics of a person. If someone cannot move, with high muscle tone, or spasticity, if they cannot eat without a gastric tube, we are used to identifying these characteristics of the body, and then we try to find solutions to make this person normal again. We have a fixed reference to what is "normal."

The hospital had given me thick folders, hundreds of pages for each child. Nowhere in any of these hundreds and thousands of pages was anything mentioned about what I experienced with Frank. There was no mention of how loving he was. There was no mention of how alert he was. Although he did not have the cognitive functions to express himself nor the motor skills, the presence of this being, his wholeness, his capacity to embrace you with his gaze, was nowhere referenced. It did not appear in those folders, and so it was not appreciated.

I knew Frank for many years after that, as a doctor. However, I must tell you, Hannah, that he also became something like my teacher. I learned that I had been meeting my patients very superficially, from an external descriptive, phenotypic approach. I had not been trained to appreciate the quality of being, and so I overlooked it. I was only looking for signs and symptoms of anything that deviated from "normal."

Frank taught me the courage, just from his being, to meet people in a much deeper, naked, transpersonal way.

I used to speak with him a lot, although he never spoke a word back to me. I was never clear if he understood the words conceptually. I could not know that. But I knew that he was present with me. He responded, he reacted. "How are you today, Frank?" I would ask him. He would show me with his body language. He would respond with a combination of movements and sounds. He would grunt when he was not feeling well. He would connect deeply and become very still when he was at ease. He had a way to communicate peace.

His parents had abandoned him, just left him at the hospital. It was too stressful for them. But the nurses who looked after him also quickly learned how to communicate with him. It was very clear when the communication was not working: he would express himself very clearly if we did not get what he was trying to say.

Question "Normal"

I remember the day he died. I cried for many days. Afterwards, he left an empty space in my life.

*

Of course, it would be an oversimplification to say that people who are disabled, mentally or physically, are healthier than normal people. But we could certainly begin to explore the possibility that some are less healthy in some ways, and also more healthy in other ways. It is just a different kind of "normal."

As I stood on that corridor, I looked to my right and saw a group of children who would soon get over their temporary illnesses, and then they would be able to go back to playing football, and win sports trophies. Later they would all grow up and make money and make everybody proud. They would do what they have been told they should do. But they may or may not be capable of real deep connection, holding someone's gaze, or feeling overwhelming gratitude.

As I looked to my left, I knew that these children in their wheelchairs would never play football. They would not even speak. But many of them had a tremendous depth of love and connection, which can be a powerful reminder to the rest of us.

Hannah, I am not suggesting that we choose one side of the corridor over the other. But I do want to remind you that we, as a society, have indeed chosen one over the other.

There were things I could give to Frank, but there was something that he gave to me. Although he was incapacitated physically, I received something immensely valuable from our exchanges. It reminded me of that which my heart constantly yearns for: a feeling of connectedness, innocence, and purity. He gave me the same nourishment that I have got at other times from being with a newborn baby, or with a dying person. It is the feeling that the struggle is over; the trying, the forcing, the contraction of individuated willpower has relaxed.

As you move through the next years you will also find your own versions of Frank. You will meet patients who challenge your idea of what is familiar and comfortable and "normal." I hope that at those times, as well as trying to support these patients to participate in the world we know, you will also allow yourself to be invited into the world that they know.

Chapter Ten
Dare to Care

Dear Hannah,

As you pass through your residency, having more contact with patients, you will be taught again and again to create and maintain a professional distance. In order to be scientific, in order to be a good doctor, you should avoid having any form of personal relationship with your patients. You can't let yourself get caught up emotionally. You will be trained, in various ways, not to get too entangled: don't create any kind of bonding. Of course, there is great benefit to these guidelines. We don't want a doctor who is performing surgery, or some other life-saving intervention, to get sentimental. This is even more clear in psychotherapy or psychiatry:

the therapist needs to be emotionally detached in order to do their job. This is simply professional.

However, there is a way to remain entirely professional in your conduct, and to also allow your heart to stay open. You can let yourself love people, and also dare to care about people. Very often, when people go to hospital, they experience that the doctor is primarily focused on statistics and data and on performing the role of a scientist. It takes courage to open your heart, and to feel love. This may not actually be your son, or your daughter, or your brother, or your sister, or one of your parents. But it is a human being with a complex human life, just like one of the people you know well and care deeply about.

Hannah, you are a woman operating in an environment that has been designed by men. Although this has changed a lot in the last few decades, medicine as we know it today was created by the masculine psyche. As a male doctor, if I approach my patients with too much heart, I may run the risk of not being taken seriously, particularly by the fathers.

It feels to me that it is time for us, particularly for your generation, to rethink some of the ways that these boundaries have been created, and to be able to establish a more open-hearted, intimate relationship with patients, while still maintaining professional boundaries. We have, in the past, seen this as a conflict. But when I talk with you, or even just think about you, I know that it is really possible for your professionalism to increase as you also allow your heart to open.

Let me tell you an inspiring story now of when one of my colleagues dared to allow his heart to open fully, and to care more deeply for one of our patients than anything I have seen before or since.

*

I was a resident, when fourteen-year-old Johann was admitted, with salmonella sepsis. The first day that I met him, he was in a single room in an old hospital. He was skinny, pale, gray and listless — it was clearly sepsis. The door was on one side of the room, and there was a big glass door on the other side, leading out to the hospital garden.

"Hey, Johann, how are you?" I asked him.

At first, Johann didn't answer me. He did not want to relate with almost any of the staff in the hospital. Finally, after a lot of waiting on my part, he said to me, "Look, I don't want to be here. I don't even know why I'm here." I told him that he was seriously ill, and that we would be ready to help him if he wanted. He told me he did not care, and did not want our help.

After about half an hour of trying to talk with him, I left the room to speak with his treating physician. Johann was HIV-positive, and my colleague had already been treating him as an outpatient for many months. Although it was available, he was not taking any HIV medication. Johann was living in an orphanage. His mother had died of AIDS, and she had also refused any medication. I discovered that he had recently attended a summer camp with the other children from the orphanage, and it was there that he had caught severe salmonella sepsis.

With all this new information, I went back to the room, together with the consultant on call, Roger. He sat on Johann's bed.

"Look, Johann," said Roger. "You may not understand fully what is going on here. We are not talking about whether you take your medication, or whether you would like to stay here or not. The question that you need to answer now, or at least within the next few minutes, is whether you want to live, or whether you want to die. If you want to live, we are here to help you. Otherwise, you are close to death." The boy responded without any hesitation.

"I want to live."

"Look," said Roger, "if that is really true, then you need to do what we recommend. Otherwise, you could be dead tonight. This is where we are."

"Fine," said Johann.

I was surprised. He had been totally blocking any communication with me. But with this other doctor, who confronted him in a much more direct way, he responded. It turns out Johann had known Roger for a long time, and trusted him.

Johann received antibiotic treatment, and he got better from the sepsis. After a few days we also started him again on anti-retroviral treatment for his HIV.

A few days later, I was sitting in my office, looking at his lab results. I did not see what I would have expected with anti-retroviral treatment. So I called Roger again.

"Roger, I just looked at Johann's charts. His hemoglobin is normal, his white cells are fine, he has no lymphocytes. His liver functions are up, but not much, and his viral count is still 50,000 copies. These results are unchanged, in spite of the anti-rets."

Roger was a consultant; he would not tell me what to do, because Johann was now under my care. He was very professional in that way. "What is your interpretation?" he asked me.

"It seems like we are not effective with the treatment," I replied. "We don't have any side effects. Do you feel he may not be taking the medication?"

"I do not 'feel' that he's not taking the medication," replied Roger, as if making little air quotes with his fingers, and smiling to me. "I know for a fact that he is not taking his drugs."

Roger came down to my office and we went back to Johann's room together. He was looking so much better, having recovered from his sepsis. But when he saw two doctors coming with great urgency, he knew something was up. He looked startled and suspicious.

"Johann, where are the pills?" Roger asked him, very directly.

"What pills?" Johann responded, acting innocent.

"Your HIV treatment. Where are the pills?"

"I'm taking them," said the boy.

"No, you are not," Roger replied, without missing a beat. "Where are they?" Johann tried to maintain his posture.

"So sorry, Johann," said Roger. "This is really important. I'm going to check everywhere." He started to open all the drawers and then to check the bed, and the pillow. Then he lifted the mattress and... boom... there they were. Six days worth of tablets. Dozens and dozens of tablets.

Johann looked completely ashamed. He shrank into himself, and he did not want to talk anymore.

"Okay, fine," said Roger. "Whatever happened, now we know that you did not take your treatment. But we need to know why."

"I don't know," mumbled the boy.

"Come on, if you want to live, we have to find out why. There has to be a good reason why you are not taking your medicine."

Roger began to offer the boy all kinds of legitimate reasons why he might not have taken the medicine. "Are you afraid of something? Are you afraid of the side effects? Do you have trouble taking them? Are there too many pills? Do you get nausea? Do you have some other kind of bad experience? Should we find a different way for you to take them?"

"No, that's not what it is... No, that's not what it is," the boy answered to each and every question.

Finally, Johann offered us the clue. "My mother also did not take her tablets," he said, almost as a justification for why it was legitimate for him to do the same.

"Aha," said Roger with a calm voice. "So you feel that you should do what your mother did?"

"Yeah," said the boy, quietly, looking down at the bed.

Slowly, we pieced it all together. He had the same disease as his mother. His mother had died. He felt guilty to take the treatment that his mother had not taken. Why should he live when his mother had died?

"You know that your mother died." Roger continued. "She could still be alive if she had taken the tablets. Do you know that?"

"Yeah. Kinda." The boy shrugged.

I started to understand. He did not want to blame his mother for having refused treatment, but he also did not want to be a traitor to her. He was in a double bind. Neither course of action seemed to be okay.

"Look," Roger continued, "if you really want to live, you have to start taking this treatment. Otherwise, this virus will kill you just the way that it killed your mother. The next salmonella, or the next bug that is going around, will be the end of you, unless we can get your immune system working again. The only way to get your immune system working is by treating this virus."

Somehow something got through to this boy that day. It was not so much what was being said. Johann had heard all this a thousand times already. It was how it was being said. Roger was not speaking to him as a detached medical observer, as he had been trained; he was speaking with great authority, like he really, truly cared. He was speaking the way that a father would speak to his son.

Johann was very silent. He was looking down at the bed, obviously struggling within himself. Then he slowly nodded his head.

"Okay," he said very quietly. But this was not the same "Okay" as before. This one was not to appease us. It came from his core.

Roger did not say anything in response. I remember this moment so well. He simply moved over to the boy, and put his hand on the teenager's knee. He looked the boy in the eye, with an unwavering gaze. There was a pin-drop silence in the room.

"Okay," Roger also finally said.

It was a decisive moment. Very few words. A deep agreement was being created "We are going to do this together."

Roger looked at me, and he nodded. We left the room together. Outside, we reflected on what had just happened in the room. Roger felt completely confident that this was all we needed. It was handled.

I went back to my office, and instructed the nurses to stay in the room whenever Johann took his pills, and to make sure he swallowed them. We would continue to measure his blood samples, to check his viral count, his liver functions, and his lymphocyte count.

Sure enough, over the next days and weeks, everything improved.

Two weeks later, he was much better. It was time for him to go back to the orphanage. Once again, I went to the room, together with Roger.

"Johann, we need to start planning that you go back to the orphanage," said Roger. "Let's talk about how we can make sure that you take your medication, once you are back there. That is going to be the key."

"Yeah. Don't worry. I will take care of it. It's fine," said the boy.

"I'm sorry, Johann," said Roger. "That's just not good enough. You need to tell me how exactly we are going to be able to check on this. We need to coordinate this with your caretaker."

"There is no need," said the boy.

"Look, I really want to make sure this happens. We are going to meet again in four weeks. I want this to be a success and not a failure." I could hear the determination and decisiveness in Roger's voice. It was palpable, in my own body.

It was obvious that Johann was very resistant and very unhappy about the prospect of going back to the orphanage. We could see his body posture shutting down, becoming more constricted. But he knew how well-intentioned Roger was; he could feel how deeply Roger wanted him to live. With Roger, he could stay open. So Johann started to speak with this doctor about how it was not easy for him to be in the orphanage, about the trip to the camp just before he came to the hospital, and how hard that had been for him.

"Tell me for real," asked Roger. His tone let the boy know that any answer was going to be all right. There was no judgment here. "Are you ready to go back to the orphanage?"

"No, I'm not," the boy replied, without hesitation. "I don't like that place at all."

"What is it about the place? Roger asked, very gently. "Is it the physical environment, or is it the people that you are most concerned about?"

"Basically, everything," said the boy.

"Do you have friends there?"

"Kinda," said the boy.

"What about your mother? Are you able to talk about your mother and your memories of her there?"

"No," said the boy.

"Would you like to talk about your mother with someone?"

"Yes. I would." Johann brightened, and sat up in the bed.

"We can surely try to find a specialist for you, in the hospital. Or do you already know someone who you would like to speak with about your mother?"

"Yes," said the boy, with more strength and certainty in his voice than I had ever heard in all these weeks. "I want to talk with you."

Roger hesitated. He glanced at me. We both knew that he was not a psychiatrist or psychotherapist, and that the hospital would not allow him to schedule time for this. "I may not have the time and space to give you what you really need," Roger said finally. I think we could both feel the sadness with which he spoke. "I am an HIV consultant. We could find a psychiatrist or psychologist to work with you." It was so obvious that the boy was very disappointed by this answer. He was crestfallen. For once in his life he had called out for what his heart wanted and needed, and he was getting a "no."

There was an uncomfortable silence.

Finally Roger broke that silence. "You know what? Why don't we meet? Outside the hospital, not in my HIV clinic, or here in the intensive care unit. Why don't we just meet someplace, and talk about your mother? Just you and me?"

We both knew, Roger and I, that this was against protocol in every possible way.

Johann visibly brightened. His eyes were suddenly shining. He was all here.

It was agreed. Johann would go back to the orphanage, after staying a little longer in the intensive care unit. Then, it was agreed that he would meet with Roger from time to time privately, as a friendship.

The boy was discharged; he was no longer under my care. I didn't think about any of this for quite a while. I met Roger about a month later. Of course, I asked Roger if he had further contact with Johann.

Roger had a wife and two sons, a little older than Johann. He explained to me that his wife was a nurse at the HIV clinic. She met Johann each time he came in for his checkups. Both of them could feel that this was not going in the right direction, and he was not going to make it alone. They spoke about Johann at home, and they agreed together to adopt him, and to make him a part of their family. Roger told me that day that Johann had already moved in with the family, and that he was doing well.

Roger and his wife did not just help Johann to take his medication, or even help him to stay alive. They gave him a completely new start on life. Johann explained to his sons, "This is Johann. He has HIV, but you do not need to be afraid. He leads a very normal life. He is not dangerous, he is just like everybody else. He just happens to have a virus, for which he is getting medication." The three boys became like normal brothers. They would sometimes all sleep in the same bed at night, and swap stories together in the dark.

Johann became fully part of the family. I never saw him again, but I did hear from Roger recently. Johann is in his late twenties now. He got a great education, and he is very successful in business. His virus is completely under control, and he is living a normal life. A happy life.

*

Obviously this is a very unusual situation. I am not suggesting that you should adopt your patients on a regular basis. You would quickly run out of room in your small apartment. But this story demonstrates that the real disease Johann was suffering from was a lack of connection, the feeling that no-one dared to care. As soon as that disease was addressed, at its roots, everything became good for him. He became whole, and he became truly healed. He did not recover from his AIDS diagnosis, but his condition became manageable, and he became a whole, happy, human being.

Although this particular solution is not something that could be easily duplicated, the important thing is that the medical system, as it still exists today, would not really think that this is the real problem. Everything is addressed at a much more superficial level.

In all his interactions with Johann (including adopting him), Roger demonstrated to me what it means to be really, truly, deeply committed to being a healer. It means that you might even go to these extremes, if you truly want to bring healing to the world, and not just be a technician who clocks in and clocks out. The commitment to wholeness is so great that it knows no boundaries. When your commitment to healing becomes greater than your commitment to just "doing a job," you learn to start looking, in every interaction, for what is underneath the presenting symptoms, just as you would with anyone you love.

Here is a story to illustrate this. When I was training as an infectious disease registrar, I worked on bone infections. I had a child come in with osteomyelitis. "Great," I said to myself. "This is good. I know everything there is to know about osteomyelitis. I'm an expert. I know how to diagnose it, I know how to treat it."

"Hey," I said confidently to the parents, "this is your lucky day. You've met the right doctor. I know how to handle this."

I went on to plan a series of tests, which included a bone marrow sample. I planned to stick a needle into the bone, suck out the bug and identify it, so I could pinpoint the right treatment for the child. I ran this by my consultant at the time, who was much more experienced.

"Yes," he said to me, "I can see where you're coming from. This is totally correct from a protocol perspective, from a scientific point of view. It is also correct from the perspective of microbiology, and infectious diseases, and antibiotic stewardship. But," the consultant went on, "I changed the way that I work since I had children of my own. You don't have kids yet. Things change once you become a parent.

"Now I ask myself," he went on, "if this was my child, would I want to put them under anesthesia, and stick a needle into the bone, and cause a wound? Now I remind myself that ninety percent of osteomyelitis cases are staphylococcus aureus. So let's just treat that. And if that doesn't work, after a few days, we can still do the bone marrow sample."

I didn't have children at that time, so it was a difficult thing for me to understand. Now that I do have children, it is much easier.

It is a very simple question, at the core of daring to care, beyond being a technician. Whatever the thing is you are planning to do, which looks like correct science, would you do this to your own child? Or any member of your own family?

In my coaching with Arjuna, he has encouraged me to start my daring to care with myself, then to let it overflow to my wife and family, and then to let it influence my work as a doctor. Here is Arjuna:

*

Hey, Hannah, Jan has just explained the very essence of daring to care. It has to start at home, in your own heart, in your own body. Once you learn how to care deeply for the needs of your own body, it becomes a training ground for being kind to all sorts of other bodies as well. It overflows at first into the way that you treat your partner, your children, your parents. It overflows into the home you share with your family, and only then it overflows into the hospital, into seeing that all beings are in some way related to you. You can choose to see people as distant from you, or you can choose to see them as close. Each choice will have a different outcome. You realize that when you are in connection, you are always at home, and you are welcoming everyone you treat into this home. Home is who you are. It is love itself.

Our deepest longing, and our deepest nourishment, is for connection. Connection with ourselves, connection with other people, connection with love itself. When that is broken, it often shows up as all kinds of physical symptoms. When we simply try to correct the symptoms with drugs and diagnostics, we frequently miss what is really going on.

Here are some tools that have proven useful in coaching others to bring forth this quality of caring.

First is to distinguish between someone's condition and who they are as a person. As a doctor, you will meet many people who appear angry, upset, and closed, just as Johann was with Jan. Whenever anyone is angry, upset, rude, or pushing you away, it is often because that person is experiencing pain and isolation. It is only hurt people who want to hurt people. If we want to learn to dare to care, we need to look right through the irritable, frightened exterior of the person and see if it is possible to connect with who they were as a child, or who they are when they are most relaxed. When someone is ill, it is often simply the disease that is talking. We have to forgive people for their grouchiness, and actively seek out their innocence, to allow ourselves to love people and to welcome them into our hearts.

Rudolf Steiner is the founder of Waldorf education. When he visited the original Waldorf cigarette factory, in Stuttgart where the first school was founded, he met with the teachers. He used to say, "When you go home at night, contemplate each of your children for a few minutes before you go to bed. Think about who they could become. Contemplate their greatest potential."

I do the same with each of my coaching clients every day, and doctors can do the same with their patients. You can think about each of your patients, and send each of them your love and your well wishes. This may not be encouraged in the contemporary medical environment, so we have to encourage ourselves to love people like they are our own children. Doctors have been trained to think that this will create attachment, or entanglement. But it does not have to. This can be a love which sets everybody free and makes everyone well.

You can start daring to care with yourself. Eating well, getting to sleep early, taking long baths, practicing meditation or yoga — these are all foundational ways to learn to dare to care for the physical body you can have more responsibility for and impact on: your own.

If you want to learn to dare to care as a doctor, you have to learn to dare to care everywhere. Care for your own body. Care for your partner. When you have children, care for them. Care for your parents. Care for your friends. Dare to care a little more than is expected of you in every environment. No exceptions. See everything as a training ground to wake up and exercise your heart.

Chapter Eleven
Create Loving Relationships

Dear Hannah,

Here is another thing that you will almost certainly hear nothing about in your training in medical school. I want to talk to you today about the very powerful connection between your effectiveness as a true healer, and the quality of your own personal relationships.

In the hospital, you learn about pathogens and antibiotics, pathophysiology and remedies. There is a learning curve; that is why you are in training: you gain professional skills and competence. Creating extraordinary loving relationships with your partner, your parents, and later with your children is also a skill you can learn and master. There are all sorts of fantastic resources available that can help you move from an adequately functional relationship to an ecstatically loving relationship. Surprisingly, this may be one of the most significant things you can do to become a truly extraordinary medical practitioner.

The reason why you have not heard about this in medical school is that your professors and doctors who have taught you, and who are going to supervise you in your residency, may be extremely accomplished and knowledgeable in treating disease, but they may not necessarily have learned the skills that create extraordinarily loving relationships. It might even be an area so weak that it becomes an embarrassment. Hence, it is not emphasized.

I don't know if you are aware of this, but the health care profession is ranking in the top six industries with the highest divorce rate and with about double the rate of suicides compared to the general population in some countries. This demonstrates that the private lives of doctors are very often out of balance. This may have something to do with long working hours, being away from home a lot, getting stressed, and then coming home frustrated or exhausted with no energy left to share. But it also has something to do with an attitude. I have already mentioned this, in my previous letters to you. The medical culture has accepted the doctor as knowledgeable, authoritative, and in certain ways superior. The patient is vulnerable, and for the medical relationship to work well, the patient must obey the doctor's prescriptions to be "compliant," as they say. This can create a kind of arrogance in medical professionals, which, if it creeps over into home life, is disastrous.

I have learned through my own crisis points in my relationships and my marriage that it is actually not so difficult to address this imbalance. It is absolutely possible to create a personal life that is so nourishing that you can feel fulfilled and complete when you arrive at the patient consultation room in the morning. This has an immeasurably powerful effect on your capacity to be an extraordinary healer.

I mentioned in a previous letter that the best practice ground you have for healing physical bodies in general is to start with the body most accessible to you: the one you inhabit and see in the mirror every morning. The next most potent training ground in becoming a heart-based physician is in attending to your relationships with the people closest to you.

Foolishly, I used to think this was not so important. In fact, I made some very unwise and naïve decisions about this area of my life, and I almost lost my marriage as a result. I simply did not understand some basic principles about deep listening, appreciation, presence, keeping my word, and transparency. As I mentioned to you earlier, my work with Arjuna started with a focus on my marriage. He helped me to remember some very simple basic principles of how to create loving relationships: things that my heart already knew, but my mind had forgotten. I was able to apply these principles first in my marriage with Jessica, then with our three children, then with my parents, then with everyone close to me, and finally... all this overflowed into my life's work as a doctor again. It creates resonance with the patients in a way that they can feel.

Later in this letter, I'm going to invite Arjuna to come online, to offer a few simple tools that you can practice in your personal relationships. But first, I want to share with you a very simple and basic insight that has made all the difference. This insight came primarily in my intimate personal relationships, but once it became clear and indisputable, I realized that it was equally true in my work as a doctor.

The word "love" can mean many things. The Greek word *agape* refers to a kind of love that is not personal. It means to love everyone, irrespective of how close or distant you are to that person. The Greek words *philia* and *storge* both mean, in different ways, to love those people close to you, whom you know well. Another kind of love is *eros*, which is connected with sexual passion. The Greeks didn't always take such a positive view of *eros*, and thought of it as sometimes dangerous, fiery, and irrational. It was, for them, the lowest form of love.

So what do we mean by the word "love" in its modern usage? It can refer to a pleasurable feeling, a subjective state of which we often crave more. Love can also refer to a way of behaving: writing poetry, sending flowers, or playing music. "Being loving" can also refer to taking actions which reflect deep caring for other people. This is the selfless love of a parent for a child. I have also come to understand love as a practice, something you can literally get better at if you apply yourself to it. And finally, through meditation or prayer or any other kind of inner work, we can come to discover love as a state of being: not so much how you behave, but who you are in your innermost self.

We, all of us, can get these different kinds of love mixed up with each other, often to our peril. I have made some big mistakes in my life in this area, and in fact learning from these mistakes and becoming clearer about what it means to be truly loving was one of the formative forces of Heart-Based Medicine.

An important distinction I had to learn was the difference between feeling love (as a pleasurable emotion) and expressing love, as speech and action, in a way that another can feel.

When it came to a beautiful young woman, expressing love often translated into a wish to become sexual, sometimes with ecstatic and sometimes with devastating consequences. Since I was a teenager, I was defining love as a subjective experience I was feeling. If my whole body was tingling with excitement and energy, if the whole world looked brighter, if I found myself spontaneously writing poems: that was love. But it often became confusing. Many times it happened that I would deeply love a girl, and think that this was the greatest love possible, but then she might tell me that she had felt disappointed, or that I did not really care for her. How could this be? I could not imagine how anyone could feel any more love than I was feeling.

I had a few girlfriends in this way when I was at medical school, sometimes having several relationships running at the same time. But then I met Jessica: tall, slim, dark-haired, and beautiful. Her big brown eyes and cheeky smile revealed her huge heart. We would meet on the riverbank after work and tell each other about our different love adventures. First a friendship and then an innocent attraction evolved between us. One sleepy Sunday morning, I woke up in her bed after a late-night summer jamboree in town. Holding her close in my arms, still half asleep, our bodies seem to have merged into one. In that moment, I knew without a doubt that this is the woman I would share my life with and build a family together.

As we built our life together, I had to learn, through deliberate and conscious practice, to recognize that love is only partly about feeling; it is much more about the effect on the other person. That has defined my relationship with Jessica since I first started this coaching: not how much love do I feel subjectively, but how much can I bring the conscious practice of love to the relationship, so that she feels opened, appreciated, lighthearted, and free. In other words, how can the quality of presence I bring to our marriage become heart-medicine that heals her from the disease of "not love," that the world so easily infects us all with. And she does the same for me.

As doctors, we have been trained that the relationship with our patients is defined by "professional conduct," by how much we have studied, how much we have learned, and how well we can apply this knowledge to solving medical conundrums.

Of course, you and I both come from healthy, loving families. We know how to be kind and nice with people, and we take this as a given. But still, the relationship with the patient is still primarily defined by a transaction of information. How can I get what I need efficiently to make an accurate diagnosis, and to prescribe the correct remedy? This can be very exciting and intellectually stimulating for anyone interested in detective work: as if every patient is a new Sudoku puzzle to be solved. And of course, patients are grateful if we do this well, because their symptoms get better. But it is a very limited version of the full potential of medicine.

When I was falling in love with girls when I was young, the relationship was all about my subjective state, even if I did not recognize it at the time. When we connect with the patient only to gather data, make a diagnosis, and then make a prescription, it can, in just the same way, become quite narcissistic and egotistical. Of course, it doesn't look that way: it looks like we are helping people altruistically. But it can also become a habit to feed the sense of being knowledgeable and powerful — unless you directly feel the limitations and the resulting helplessness and frustration.

At home, my closest relationships have become defined by what I can give: by the well-being and happiness of the other person. This does not create the same kind of euphoric endorphin-induced rush of romantic feelings that "falling in love" used to: instead it leads to a calm, centered, peaceful relaxing into being a loving person. Just the same thing can happen with patients: it requires a deep curiosity and caring about their well-being in a multidimensional way, and recognizing that the diagnosis of conditions and prescription of treatments is only one part of that.

I can clearly recognize this difference now by how I feel at the end of each consultation, and how I feel at the end of the day. When I used to show up for work simply to be a professional, and to do my job in a somewhat clinical but also distant way, I used to feel drained at the end of the day. I would bring that exhausted feeling home, and then I had nothing to give to my beloved and the children. When I open my heart as a doctor, and really allow myself to care for people, as one human being to another, I feel energized and inspired, and I can bring that home to the family. Then our life at home is also nourishing and energizing, and I can bring that fullness also to my work. This used to be "random," and only recently did I learn to consciously live and work like this. The love I have learned to generate and amplify in my personal relationships feeds my work as a doctor, and deliberately practicing as a doctor with an open heart means I have more to give to my family.

Often, we think of the work-life balance as a question of balancing time: how many hours should I spend at work versus how many hours do I devote to family time? This is definitely something that needs attention, but it is also not simply a matter of how you devote your time. You can deliberately choose to practice a disposition which creates an overflow of well-being, both at home and at work. What looks like a dilemma or a conflict to solve between personal and professional life can actually become synergistic: they feed and support each other.

*

Let me tell you a little story about how this can work in practice. It would be very easy for you to duplicate this anytime. This story is about Naima, my youngest daughter, but this would equally apply with anyone from your life: your father or your mother, your boyfriend, or anyone whom you really love and know that they love you too.

It was a Monday morning, and everyone was in Monday-morning mode. The ward was full, six patients were waiting in the emergency unit waiting for admission. Stress levels were running high; we needed to discharge six or eight patients to make space for the new ones. The nurses were all rushing around, very busy. The residents were feeling overwhelmed, having to absorb information about new patients they had never met. I am sure you know this feeling already.

Then one of the residents called me to attend to a difficult patient. It was a small child, very sick, and the father was extremely upset. He did not feel heard, and did not feel that the medical issues of his child were really being acknowledged. They were back in the hospital for the fourth time in three weeks, with a series of different medical issues. The father was behaving very aggressively with the nurses, so they called me in. "This man needs a senior physician to put him in his place," said the nurse, "and to set the record straight. We are doing all that we can." I was ready to confront the father, as I have a zero tolerance for aggression against hospital staff.

Then... I remembered.

I remembered my initial calling to be a doctor. I remembered why I was here. I remembered everything that I had learned by practicing love at home.

I asked the nurse to excuse me, and I stepped aside for a moment from the bustle of the hospital. I closed my eyes, and I deliberately remembered something that had happened the night before:

*

I have just come home. I open the door, and Naima runs toward me, jumps up into my arms. She is so happy that I am home from work. "Daddy... Daddy..." She is wearing little leggings, with roses printed on them, and a little dress on top. Her hair is gathered on each side in plaits, like Pippi Longstocking, and they are flapping like wings as she runs toward me. She raises her arms up for me and yells, "My best daddy is home." She hugs me very firmly, and makes deep gurgling sounds. "Hmmmm... hmmmm... hmmm... I missed you so much, my best daddy. You are the best of all daddies."

"I missed you too. You are the best of all Naimas."

"You are my favoritest daddy in the whole world."

"You are my favoritest Naima in the whole world."

Then there are no words anymore. We are just holding each other, and feeling this love, for several minutes. Suddenly, she lifts her head from my shoulder, and says "Daddy, come. Come, Daddy, I need to show you something." She takes me to see a painting she has made: a painting of Naima and her daddy. My tears are rolling...

I opened my eyes again, in the hospital. It had only taken one or two minutes to activate that memory. I stepped into the room, which was quite chaotic. The father was in panic, pacing around. The child looked very uncomfortable, lying awkwardly on the bed. I walked toward the father, very slowly, still carrying the feeling in my chest from this memory. I moved toward him, and immediately saw through the layer of worry and aggression to recognize him as a loving, concerned man, who had understandable worry about his child.

He sensed this immediately. Now he was not being met by an official from the hospital, he was being met by another father, another man who also cherishes his child. His whole behavior changed. He seemed temporarily disoriented. He could feel that this was a different kind of energy walking into the room. It took him a couple of minutes to change gears. I saw the exhaustion and the terror in his eyes. At the beginning, his mind was still running at a million thoughts a minute. "This thing is happening... and this thing is happening... and this is happening, and no one is listening to me."

I listened. That is all I did. I did my best to radiate and to send him the love that I had generated in my chest from the memory with my own daughter. Slowly, the speed of his talking slowed down. There were more gaps between the sentences. For five minutes, I didn't say anything. Then, finally, I simply said "I can completely understand your concern. I am totally with you. Let's look at this together, and let's find a solution together. What is it that you need the most right now? What is it that you believe is really going on? What are your greatest fears?"

This young father felt deeply heard, he felt deeply seen, and he was quiet. We sat down together. I suggested that he take his child into his arms, as we spoke together. His child also became quiet, more comfortable. We didn't talk about any of the things that he thought the residents or the nurses had done wrong. I just listened to him, and we focused on his needs. Then we made a plan together, one that we created together and that we agreed upon. We followed the plan, he was happy, he felt heard, and all was good.

The whole situation changed, simply by remembering a moment from my life at home, by bringing some of the gold dust from my home life into the hospital, carrying that gently in my heart.

When people are upset, and in a panic, it may seem like they need advice, or strategy, or technique. But I have come to understand that the most immediate and primary need people have in these situations is to be heard, and seen, and understood. This is something very simple, very human.

The more that you can practice this at home, outside of the hospital, the more it will be accessible, as your state of being, with your patients. You are providing them with the space of healing in your heart,. But first, you must open the space within yourself, and the best place to do this is at home.

I learned some very simple skills in those first months of coaching with Arjuna, which cultivate this kind of space. Now I'm going to ask him to describe a few of them to you.

*

Hey, Hannah. Of course, we don't have space in this little book to go into this in all the detail that I did with Jan. So I will simply label for you five basic principles that are very easy to integrate, and which will transform relationship most quickly into a practice ground for the kind of love that can overflow into your practice as a doctor. If you would like to go more deeply into exploring any of these principles as practices at home, we have included a link to the Heart-Based Medicine site that you can follow.

Commitment. We often think of commitment as allegiance to one particular person. This is the principle behind "till death do us part." In fact, it can be very difficult to maintain that kind of commitment. Relationships change in all kinds of unpredictable ways, and it may not always be possible to guarantee that you will stay with the same one person forever. But you can commit to love. You can commit to being the most loving version of yourself, no matter how the outward story changes. If you share that commitment to love together with your partner, or in fact with anyone you are close to, you can support each other in the practice of love. A simple practice is to make a ritual of commitment in this way, which I have shared with you in the link below.

Deep listening. When we become really curious about the other person, when we really want to know what they are feeling and thinking underneath what we see on the surface, we focus less on trying to change the other person to accommodate our needs, and we become more of a loving presence. One way to explore this is through the practice called "Deep Listening," which is also accessible from the link below.

Appreciation. Thought processes get activated when it seems like there is something to be fixed. You could say that the mind is simply a problem-solving machine. Hence, we often communicate the things that we don't like, things that we want to change, but we don't necessarily speak about the things that are wonderful and marvelous. Just like the plants in your garden, the ones that you water will flourish and blossom. Experiment with a playful game of expressing at least five appreciations each day to your partner, or to someone close to you. "I really appreciate how beautiful you make things look. I appreciate how kind and attentive you are."

Honesty. We often interpret honesty as telling the factual truth about stories that happened in the past. Sometimes that may be useful. But there is also another kind of honesty, which has a magical effect. This kind of honesty is oriented to what is happening in the present moment: to align your speaking with your subjective experience. It doesn't do much to feed our minds, but it creates immediate intimacy. In the link below I've shared with you a simple practice you can adopt in just a few minutes a day which will dramatically increase your capacity to be honest, vulnerable, and intimate.

Humor. Relationships of all kinds suffer from getting too serious and intense, and flourish when there is an atmosphere of humor and fun. Of course, when things get a little sticky and tense, humor can feel forced. But there is a simple game you can play, which is easy to pick up, which can turn the most awkward and tense areas of any relationship into the ones that make us laugh the most. I've also included guidelines for that practice in the link below.

If you'd like to experiment with these practices that you can integrate at home right away, please follow this little link: heartbasedmedicine.org/registerbook

Chapter Twelve
Believe in Healing Potential

Dear Hannah,

When we work in a hospital, we are trained to be empirical. We look at data to diagnose, and treat disease and to predict health outcomes with accuracy. In this way of seeing things, feelings of optimism or intention are not encouraged, as they are seen to cloud seeing data objectively.

If you wish to be truly empirical, you must simply look at the test results, and then compare them with as many similar test results from the past as are available. An empiricist might say, "Statistically speaking, if we look historically at people who have had similar test results to yours, there is a ninety-seven percent chance that you will be dead within a month." This is not something you would ever want to say to someone. However, to be truly empirical, it is necessary to look at the data without any perceptual bias, or any attempt to influence it. Therefore, there is no place in empiricism for intention, or prayer, or wishing the best for someone.

There is another way to meet your patients: where you actually wish them well. You have intention. You would really like to see this person get better. If this was a child in the hospital, and the mother or father heard that there is a ninety-seven percent chance that the child will die, then as long as that child is still alive today, most parents focus on the three percent chance that the child will live. As long as there is any small chance of getting better, the eyes of love will focus entirely on that. The eyes of hope, the eyes of inspiration, the eyes of intention, the eyes of the heart, will always focus on the intended outcome, rather than the statistically likely probability.

In the world of the heart, intention is key. Wishing someone well is the language that the heart speaks.

Doctors are thoroughly trained in how to be empirical and scientific: to not give anyone false hope, to be skeptical. A doctor today is more of a scientist and a statistician than a mystic. Even a hundred years ago medicine was still frequently practiced within the realms of religion: where the power of prayer, the mercy of God, and divine intervention were all included as parts of the puzzle.

We all have to decide what is the most healthy balance of these two ways of being present with patients. A radiologist is taught to look at the results of a CT scan and to make an objective diagnosis. Very often, the radiologist who does this work never meets the patient at all. The results of the test and the interpretation are passed on to the patient through someone else. On the other hand, the deeply religious or spiritual mother of a sick child will think only in terms of miracles. She believes that anything becomes possible with the grace of something beyond the human mind that we do not understand,

As a doctor, over the years I have learned to integrate a balance of these two ways of viewing my patients. In addition to prescribing tests and reading the results, I have also learned to deeply believe in the healing potential of my patients, sometimes against all odds. I do not require my patients to comply with statistical norms. Where there is deep intention, when there is hope, when there is the loving support of a community, miracles become more and more what we can hope to expect.

Let me tell you about one of my patients who, very early in my career, taught me about the miraculous power of intention.

*

Before I started medical school, I worked as a home nurse for a private company. One day, they sent me to an apartment about twenty kilometers outside of Zürich. I had to climb the stairs to the tenth floor. A woman in her mid-forties answered the doorbell; she looked pale and exhausted. She explained that I was here to look after her son, who was almost completely paralyzed, lying in a hospital bed in the apartment. Very shortly, she had to go to work.

I entered the room. A young man was lying in the bed, with his upper body tilted up by the bed. He had very short hair, and the lines on his young face let me know that he had recently lost a lot of weight. He had a hole in his windpipe, which was clearly how he had previously been receiving breathing support when in hospital.

He looked at me with curiosity. I pulled up a chair, and sat next to him. Although he couldn't move, his eyes were very alive, curious and open. I introduced myself, and reached out my hand. Then I realized he had great difficulty even lifting his arm. So I extended my hand even further, to touch his.

"Hi. My name is Jan. I am here to take care of you. How are you?"

He looked at me; I could see from his eyes that he was trying to speak, but he could not say anything. In just that first morning, I discovered that we would have to find another way to communicate, through other routes. The hole in his throat had a little plug, which he could insert in order to speak, but then he had to remove it again to breathe before uttering the next word.

Just that first morning, we started to develop a system. First, we agreed upon finger signals for "yes" and "no." Later we agreed that closing his eyes would mean "no," and opening his eyes a little bigger would mean a "yes." Like this, I could do all the talking, asking him questions, and he could simply answer yes or no. He made it absolutely obvious that he desperately wanted to be in connection and communication.

I went on working with him regularly in this apartment for four to six months. I used to cook for him, and then spoon feed him the food. He could have only puréed meals, so I put it all in the blender, and then brought it to him as a mush. He loved minced meat, and potato purée. Sometimes, it was difficult for him to eat, and to manage to swallow. Then he would cough violently, and I would have to take a catheter and put it down his airways to suck out phlegm, sometimes mixed with potato purée from his windpipe.

He had tremendous motivation and power to recover his autonomy. I brought him paper and colored pens, and he learned to communicate very clumsily through drawing and painting. I brought an alphabet board, and he learned to spell out words by pointing at the letters. He learned to tell me his name: D...A...V...I...D... He learned to put his finger over the tracheostomy, and to close it, so he could attempt to speak words. He could put pressure on his vocal cords. Over these months, his language skills became much better. He was working with a speech therapist, and he was able to speak more and more words. I was helping David with absolutely everything: brushing his teeth, washing, bathroom needs, everything. He became like my younger brother.

I totally loved this man. There were pictures on the wall from his time when he was fit and well and having fun as a teenager. Slowly, he was able to explain to me that while in the army he had an acute episode of meningitis. He obviously wanted to tell me more about this, so I asked him questions, and he responded in the way we had established: closing the eyes for a "no," and opening the eyes wide for "yes."

"So you were in the intensive care unit?" Big eyes.

"For how long?" On the alphabet board: two months.

Slowly, he was able to explain that he had a tube down his throat for breathing, and another tube down his nose to empty his stomach. He had a catheter in his penis to empty his bladder. A central catheter in his neck. He had peripheral lines in his hands, and he was hooked up to every kind of monitoring device the hospital could offer. He could not move at all when he was in intensive care; he could not speak, or even open his eyes.

But he could hear.

"So David, what could you do at this point?" He just looked at me, and shrugged his shoulders.

"Not much at all, right?" He made a grimacing face.

"You couldn't do anything, or even communicate with people?" Now he opened his eyes very wide. He started to get more and more agitated, and to move his whole body in the bed. He was clearly remembering something very difficult.

"Is there a specific memory that you want to tell me about?"

Tears welled up in his eyes.

"David," I said. I took his hand. "Did something happen? Was there something specific that happened that makes you cry now when you remember it?"

Through this very slow communication, he let me know about a particular time when he heard a group of people speaking next to his bed, talking about him. It was the doctors, talking with his parents, explaining to them that they did not predict he would ever wake up again. Probably, they said, he is just like a vegetable now. He is probably brain dead.

"Wow. You could hear this?" His eyes went big again. Now, he was getting much more energized and excited. His whole body was involved.

"So how did you feel?"

He struggled this time to put pressure on his throat, to make sound. "Fuck... No... I... Will... Survive." The power and life force streaming out of him now was extraordinary. He taught me the meaning of the word "survivor."

I used to drive each day to his house in my old white VW bus. It had previously been a butcher's van that I had completely refurbished. Outside, it was plain and white. Inside, I had installed a bed, and benches, and all kinds of beautiful things. I had herbs hanging from the ceiling that I had picked and were drying. Whenever I told David about my bus, a look of both longing and excitement spread over his face.

One day, I could see that we had made tremendous progress with his physical skills. Before, I would put the cup to his lips. Now, he wanted to help me. Before, I was spoon-feeding him. Now, he wanted to hold the spoon and let me help him. Anything and everything that was remotely on the edge of being possible, he wanted to do. He had a device that helped him practice standing up. He worked extremely hard at it. His willpower to get better was unbelievable. He was willing to go to the extremes of what his body would allow him to do.

One day, when I arrived at his house, I knew that it was time.

"David, you know what? It's a beautiful day outside today. I am here with my van. We have become best friends. You know what I would love to do today? I would love to go to the lake with my best friend. Are you in?"

His body exploded with energy. He was chuckling, and coughing, and completely enjoying himself. I did have a license to transport disabled people in Germany, but not in Switzerland, and certainly my car was neither suited nor licensed for this. So it was a risk. His willpower and determination to break the limits of what was possible was irresistibly infectious. I saw his overwhelming joy that there could be a chance to get out of this small room and see real life again.

"We have just a few hours to do this, so let's make it our project together. We are going to go to the lake, and then will have to also get home again."

It took about an hour for us to get ready and prepare everything. He showed me everything we would need. He pointed to the different devices we should take. He had a special attachment for his wheelchair to allow him to go up and down stairs. Luckily, at that time I was physically strong, so everything worked smoothly, and we made it down to the street.

I had planned to put him in the wheelchair in the back of the van, but that did not work. With all the modifications I had made, the wheelchair would not fit. But now there was no looking back. I lifted him out of the wheelchair, and into the passenger seat into the front of the van, and fastened his seatbelt. The wheelchair was stored in the back.

And then, there we were. He was almost screaming with joy and gesturing wildly throughout the drive. "Hungh!!… Aaaaaaaauuugh!!… Yaaaaw!!…" He was making noises as loudly as he could, and insisted that both windows were open. I had long dreadlocks at that time. What a pair we must have seemed to the other Swiss motorists.

We arrived at a beautiful lake outside of Zürich, with a small island in the middle. We parked the van. I pulled the wheelchair up next to his door, helped him out and into his wheelchair. We were laughing and joking all the time. I pushed him in his wheelchair through the meadow, until we were just next to the waterside. Then I took off his socks and shoes, folded up the supports, so he could touch the ground with the soles of his feet. The intense pleasure he took in this was palpable.

David's face was flooded with relaxation and joy. Old memories were being reawakened in his body. Then I propped him up against a tree, so he could recline there and enjoy the view, and the afternoon.

Finally, we had to do the whole process in reverse. We had to wheel him back to the van, get him back into the seat, and drive back through the town. We got him back into the wheelchair, very slowly up the stairs, into the apartment, and back into his bed. He was completely radiant and fulfilled.

Soon after our trip to the lake, I had to go back into military service; at the time, there was no alternative to this in Switzerland other than prison. About nine months later, I worked for this company again, and they asked me if I was willing to go back to him. Of course, I said yes.

By this time, David could speak again. He still had the tube in his throat, but it would soon be removed. Immediately, he wanted to re-enact that scene in our minds together: the day we went to the lake. He was so appreciative, cherishing those fond memories.

After this I went to live in England to continue my studies. When I came back to Switzerland, I discovered that he had moved to Majorca. That had always been his dream. There is a village in Majorca for disabled people. He got some kind of disability insurance, and set his heart on saving enough to buy a house there.

That was David's spirit. He looked for what seemed impossible, and then he set his heart on it. He refused to be part of someone's probability statistics.

*

When I told this story to Arjuna, he asked me if this was an isolated incident, or if I could recognize the same quality: of seeing the healing potential in people, with other patients as well. As I reflected upon this question, I realized how important it is to ask our patients what they see as their potential.

I have been surprised to discover that not everybody really wants to be whole and healthy, at least not with all of themselves. For example, someone may really want to stop coughing, but they may not be motivated to stop smoking cigarettes. Someone could be very obese due to their eating behavior and understand the health risks that come with it. You can visualize that person losing weight, and being fit and happy. But your patient may not share your vision. Eating a lot of sweet, sticky food may be a higher priority for that person than how you think it should be.

Arjuna shared with me that in this way the work of a doctor is very similar to the work of a coach. Here, let me hand you over to him now.

*

Hannah, when my children were young, I wanted to find a really visionary school where they could grow and prosper. I went to visit our local charter school, which had been founded along the principles laid down by Rudolf Steiner, founder of Waldorf education. The first time I went to the school, before my children were enrolled, I could not restrain myself from crying, I was so touched by what I saw in the classrooms. The seventh-grade teacher was sitting — not at his desk but on his desk — leading a conversation with his class about democracy. These were twelve- and thirteen-year-olds, but the teacher had such a palpable respect for and curiosity about their opinions. He was using the educational process to draw out the children's wisdom.

Rudolf Steiner used to ask his teachers, at the original Waldorf school, created for the employees of the Waldorf-Astoria cigarette factory in Stuttgart, to perform a little visualization each night. He asked the teachers to think of each child for a few moments before going to sleep. He asked them to reflect upon the highest possibility of that child: the greatest they could accomplish; the peak of love and creativity, happiness, and service they could contribute. When teachers are willing to do it, it helps to make them truly great.

As a doctor, you can cultivate the same quality of envisioning your patient's most healed potential. Perhaps you can remember sometimes, at the end of the day, to see each patient not as sick, but to see them in their full potential as healthy and whole.

It is also important to ask your patients what they see as their potential. Of course, it is important to acknowledge people's suffering, and to reassure each person that you understand what they are experiencing, and that you are committed to finding the best available treatments. But it is also very important to listen to however they see themselves in the future.

All of this is about starting with the person in front of you, and then following that person in the direction they genuinely want to go.

Sometimes, this means you have to take slower, smaller steps to reach an achievable goal. The intuition of the patient may be more modest, but for that person it may feel more achievable. What you see for them might be too big a step, or too far from where they are at the moment.

Like this, you and your patient set up a collaborative, mutually respectful relationship, a shared understanding of what the condition is they are suffering from, how it feels to be living inside a body that has this condition, and also the goal of the healing process, including all of the sacrifices and discipline that may be required to achieve that.

Chapter Thirteen
Set the Tone for the Day

Dear Hannah,

As you may have noticed in previous letters, I've had an up-and-down relationship with taking care of my body. There have been times when I have taken extremely good care of myself, and I have been very healthy. There were other times when I let it slip.

Just like you, I grew up in a very healthy family, in the countryside, where I got plenty of exercise and great local food. We always had fresh meat and vegetables from local organic farmers. The dark red sweet tomatoes plucked from the plant tasted like real tomatoes and the young carrots pulled from the sun-warmed soil will always be my reference for what a carrot can taste like. I got plenty of time outdoors in the fresh air. So it was in my blood from a young age how to take good care of myself. Even when I was a teenager and playing drums in a jazz band, I still loved to cook well, and to make teas and tinctures from wild herbs that I gathered.

Later, there were periods when I pushed my body too hard, particularly during my student days. Working for exams, I learned to live on black coffee and junk food, treating myself with a cigarette during breaks. I would even go for days without sleep when I was working in a challenging surgical firm. But then it didn't take too long before I took a job in India, and I found my balance again. I got up early in the morning and went to bed early in the night. I took time for stillness, and I got training in the ancient practices and diet of Ayurveda. It has been for me like this throughout my life. I get out of balance for a while, but then something happens, either a decision from inside myself or a change of environment, and I return to the health and balance that I grew up with as a child.

I was at a low point in this pattern when I decided to get coached, as I described to you in my first letter. By this point, I was working as a vaccine-safety specialist for the Brighton Collaboration, and I was traveling frequently, in addition to my clinical duties at the University Children's Hospital. I would travel to conferences around the world about vaccine safety. For business meetings, in Europe, I would leave Basel late at night, stay over in a hotel, and get back the next evening. I would regularly fly overseas to places like the Centers for Disease Control in Atlanta, the Bill & Melinda Gates Foundation in Seattle, or at the National Institutes of Health just outside Washington, D.C. to meet with outstanding colleagues. I would arrive late afternoon, check into the hotel, start immediately with the first meeting until late at night, get up again at 4:30 a.m., with the help of jet lag and preparing the day's meeting. I could do this for several days, and then fly back again on the night flight to Switzerland, be back at the hospital early morning, and work in clinics the same day full on until the evening. I lived like this for many years, completely dedicated to furthering the cause of safer vaccines and transparent communication about them based on rigorous science.

It seems that I have a body that can operate in this way. It will go for weeks on end with just three or four hours of sleep, and I still seem to remain functional, albeit with the help of light food and lots of coffee.

This was the kind of rhythm I was in when I realized that things had to change. I was able to function, but that was about it. By pushing myself so hard, I had lost my spark, I had lost my connection with my heart.

Initially, I had a lot of resistance to working with a coach. I didn't want someone else telling me what to do with my life. I'm a medical doctor, thank you very much, and I know plenty about how to take care of bodies. But soon, I discovered that coaching is not about someone telling me what to do. It is more about someone asking me the right questions, with curiosity, so I can reconnect with my own wisdom. In fact, it is very similar to what works best with patients, when the doctor is truly curious and has some humility.

Early on in that coaching relationship, we were able to review all the things I ha done in the past that allowed me to be at my best. Arjuna taught me a few new tricks: like the practice of Qi Gong to circulate energy through the body. Mostly, he helped me in pulling out some good habits from my closet, where they had been gathering dust, brushing them off and then putting them back into action. Within a few weeks, we were able to re-create a daily routine to start the day. It did not take me long to reconnect with how it had been in India for the first hour or two of the day. It became clear to me that how you spend these early morning hours determines the quality of the rest of the day that follows.

Now I wake up every day at least one hour before the dawn, long before the rest of the family is awake. I drink a glass of warm lemon water, and then I sit with my eyes closed for 30 or 40 minutes, followed by about the same amount of time spent circulating energy through my body, using Qi Gong. Finally, I set some intentions for my day. I think not only about the things I want to get done, but also about the way that I want to do them, and the kind of person I want to be.

Now, it seems very strange to think back to my old way of living where I would jump out of bed at the last minute, throw back a quick coffee, hardly speak to my family, and rush off at high speed to the hospital. I understand now that it is just like surgery. Before you go in to operate on someone, you scrub up. Even before you go into meeting a patient for a consultation, you disinfect your hands. It is basic procedure. In just the same way, I learned to clean up my consciousness, my state of mind, and how I feel, before I am ready to meet people.

Now I will hand you over to Arjuna, and he will tell you about some of the guidelines he has found helpful in supporting people to develop a good morning routine.

*

Hi, Hannah. It's me again. What Jan describes as a busy medical doctor is not so unusual. I hear exactly the same thing from executives, from solo entrepreneurs, from activists and filmmakers and just about everybody else. Even the people who write books and teach seminars and offer coaching around well-being often succumb to the same story: "I just don't have enough time for daily practice." I often ask people the same set of questions, and it seems to help.

"I understand that you are very busy," I say. I get an enthusiastic response.

"You probably find that you don't have enough time to take care of yourself as you would like to." Another big nod.

"You probably even find that you are cutting back on sleep to be able to get it all done." Another big yes.

"I can imagine that there must be days when you are so busy that you just jump out of bed, still in the clothes you were sleeping in, or even wearing nothing at all, and then you run out of the house without brushing your teeth, or taking a shower or brushing your hair, and you go straight to work." At this point, I cease to get the affirmative response. No one has agreed that it goes this far.

No matter how busy it gets, everyone says they always have enough time to take a shower, to brush their teeth, to brush their hair, get dressed in some nice clothes. Breakfast? Maybe not. So then I simply ask: how come you have time for the shower, and the clothes, and the teeth and the hair, but not for other ways to prepare yourself for the day? Everyone laughs. "This is just a matter of basic standards," they say. "You cannot go to work in your nightclothes, or without washing yourself. People would be offended."

This is actually quite correct. If you were to show up without a shower or brushing your teeth, it would offend people's noses. If you showed up at work without brushing your hair, or putting on some nice clothes, it would offend their eyes. This is a matter of basic values. Taking time in the morning to prepare yourself for the day is just a matter of shifting your "set point" of what you think is adequate preparation before you are fit for the world.

Skipping basic morning routine tasks would offend people's senses. But in just the same way, if you don't have a way to prepare your consciousness and your emotions, you may offend people in other ways, by acting stressed or insufficiently sensitive to other people's needs and emotions.

During the night you have been dreaming. All sorts of strange things may have been happening. In the morning, you need to prepare to be the best version of yourself. A morning practice is a way to deliberately and consciously open your heart, and to reconnect with the source of love.

This is something we can choose to do every day. It is just the same with the kitchen. If you clean your kitchen, you can't just do this once a year, and that's it. You have to clean the kitchen every time you use it, if you want it to stay clean.

This is very easy to set straight, as Jan suggested above. If you take just a few weeks, or a month, to integrate a few simple practices, quickly they become second nature. Then you would not dream of going out of the house without first putting yourself into the best possible state, in every way.

Here are some of the components which make the most difference when people reflect on what would make a great morning routine. This is not a one-size-fits-all formula. Take these as gentle suggestions to experiment with. Be creative, and see what works for you: for your temperament, and your body, and your lifestyle. Jan tells me that this is not taught in medical school: to prepare yourself at the beginning of the day to become the best version of yourself. So it is something you will have to bring from your side.

We have collected together some resources that you can check into when you have time that will guide you into each of these practices in more detail. You and your friends can simply go to heartbasedmedicine.org/ registerbook and you get immediate access to everything we have prepared for you. You can tell your friends that this is a gift.

Wake up early

If you are going to prepare yourself for the day, it's best to do it early in the morning, if possible before dawn. Of course, this depends on your schedule at the hospital. You have undoubtedly heard the old wives' tale that an hour of sleep before midnight is worth two hours after. We have a lot of historical evidence to back that up. It's easy to forget that electricity has only been available in domestic homes for less than 100 years. Prior to that, all of our ancestors, for more than 250,000 years, went to sleep soon after the sun went down, and then woke up before the sun had risen. I encourage everyone to at least experiment with getting back in touch with this "circadian rhythm." Initially, it might feel a little strange and antisocial to not be available for late evening dinners anymore. You can always make occasional exceptions, and you can go dancing till 2 a.m. every once in a while. But the rest of the time, going to bed as early as your schedule at the hospital will allow, and then waking up naturally, without an alarm clock, before the dawn, is one of the shifts in lifestyle that will most powerfully increase your sense of well-being and allow you to become more present, focused, and connected.

Drink lemon water

As Jan mentioned, many people who have experimented with a morning practice report that drinking a glass of warm water with a whole lemon squeezed into it first thing in the morning stimulates your liver, and wakes your body up for the day. You can also add a small pinch of sea salt. This is a great time to also take mineral supplements as needed.

Sit Doing Nothing

The most powerful and effective thing that we can do to change the quality of the day and to make the greatest contribution to others is actually not a thing at all. It is taking time for no thing. After you wake up, sit on the bed or in the chair and close your eyes. It may be easier for you to purchase a blindfold (I like the one made by Tempur that you can buy on Amazon).

Then just sit, and observe, and wait.

You don't need to learn any fancy meditation techniques or special breathing or visualizations or anything. If you just sit and observe the thoughts that are passing, the emotional fluctuations, and the sensations in your body, with a relaxed and detached curiosity, they start to settle down on their own. Then it is as though a kind of perfume gets released. Slowly, after some time you feel less caught up in the thoughts and feelings and body sensations, and you relax more into *being* that which is observing. Instead of consciousness being something you experience, you know that it is who you are. People quickly discover that it is peaceful, relaxed, and inherently loving.

In the resources we mentioned above, there is a guided audio, as an MP3 audio file, which can remind you how simple and intuitive this practice can be.

Move Energy

This is also a very effective practice that people report dramatically changes their day. There are lots of ways to do this. Some people prefer a more "masculine approach" using Qi Gong movements that were developed by Shaolin monks in China thousands of years ago. These practices were initially developed by men for men, which is why we could say they are a little more masculine in their style.

A lot of women say that a more feminine approach that suits them better is simply to put on some music and then take some time to move. This is not a kind of formal dancing like the Salsa or the Waltz. It is more a question of "being danced," allowing the music to move your body.

Either way, whether it's Qigong or dance or walking or jumping on a trampoline, anything which frees up energy will allow you to feel more flexible and relaxed during the day.

Set Intentions

Finally, before you end your morning practice and get on with your day, we suggest you take a few minutes with a journal and a pen to set your intentions for the day.

Maybe you already know some of the patients you will be seeing. What do you hope to accomplish with them?

Maybe there are certain patients or colleagues who have proven to be a challenge for you in the last days.

What kind of disposition do you want to bring when you meet?

How do you want to take care of yourself today? Maybe you want to remember to take a real break at a certain point or to eat a proper lunch.

Finally, you can write one or more lines about who you want to be today. What kind of a person do you want people to experience you as?

Chapter Fourteen
Learn from Mistakes

Dear Hannah,

When you are feeling stressed all day, moving between patients, with fifteen-minute appointments, when there is a backlog of patients, and the feeling of always rushing, you inevitably move into high-performance mode. As we know, this is characterized by dominance of the sympathetic nervous system. Your brain will be running on the neurotransmitters associated with stress rather than relaxation, with more adrenaline and steroids flowing in the blood. You are in emergency mode.

We already know that when there is more sympathetic nervous system dominance, there will be a suppression of parasympathetic nervous system activity. This means that if you need to go to the bathroom, you will hardly notice it. If your eyes are itchy, because you need to go to sleep, you ignore it. If you are hungry, or achy, or have any other kinds of messages from the body, they get ignored, because they are inconvenient and it is necessary to get the job done. Whenever you are in emergency, you cannot afford to think about what your body needs in this moment.

Not only does your body suppress biological messages about the bathroom or food or the need to lie down, but equally emotional messages also get pushed aside. Anything that might cause you to feel self-doubt or self-reflection will be deflected. If you are working on someone to try to save their life, you can't afford to stop and ask yourself, "Is there something I'm missing here? Am I being insensitive?" It is hard to monitor yourself carefully for making mistakes when you have an emergency to deal with.

If you suppress messages from the parasympathetic nervous system for too long, they tend to build up and then pour out all at once. If you keep ignoring them, day after day, you can become arrogant and defensive. This is why it is so important at the end of the day to stop for a few minutes, and to just listen.

Learn from Mistakes

At the beginning, you will listen to your body. What does it have to tell you? "I'm tired. I'm hungry. I need to pee." Then you may also discover feelings as well. "I'm sad. I feel hopeless." You may discover feelings of regret, even feelings of shame or remorse for how you did not live up to your values in the day.

Having a time at the end of the day when you can reflect upon things is a great way to listen to all of these messages which have been pushed aside when you were busy, busy, busy.

I want to tell you a story today about a time when I finally came to listen to those messages, and it has made me a better doctor ever since.

*

It was 11 o'clock in the morning on a Thursday. I was working at St George's Hospital in London in the accident and emergency department. Two girls came in; they were obviously Afro-Caribbean. They were both wearing very colorful clothes, as is common to that culture. The younger girl was about eleven years old, pre-puberty. She had very short black hair, and a very thin, slender body. The other girl was only a few years older, perhaps fifteen or sixteen. Her black curly hair was gathered up and bound in a cloth on top of her head. As was quite customary in that part of

London, it was clear that they had dressed up for the hospital, and they wanted to make a good impression. Prior to working in London, I would have been surprised when a young child would come in with a sibling, but I had come to realize that it was quite common there. Both parents would be working, and the older children would take care of the younger children when they had to go to the hospital and needed to spend many hours there.

The younger girl was sitting on a stretcher, with her arms stabilizing her chest like a tripod behind her back to try to open her airways to help her breathe. She could hardly finish a complete sentence, as she was so short of breath. Her sister was standing next to her, holding her and supporting her, and answering questions on her behalf. I examined the younger girl. She had a racing heart rate and she was clearly stressed; her breathing was very labored, rapid, and wheezy. Her sister told me that this was the first time she had these symptoms. Nothing like this had happened before. There were no triggers or risk factors for asthma. She didn't have a respiratory tract infection. She had no known allergies. She had no exposure to smoke, or dust, pets, or extreme cold. Because it was April, I assumed that this must be a reaction to pollen. It was the only explanation I could imagine, that she was having an asthmatic reaction.

The older girl was extremely nervous about the poor condition of her younger sister. She was talking very fast, trying to explain that she did not understand how her sister could suddenly have such difficulty breathing, out of the blue.

I firmly believed, because of the breathing pattern, that this was an acute asthma attack. I gave her medication to inhale that she could use to open her airways. She took the medicine, and improved quite quickly. They stayed in the accident and emergency department for a few hours, and then she got so much better that I felt comfortable sending them home, with a diagnosis of acute asthma and the appropriate treatment. I did not do any further tests. On that morning it was a very full unit, and I felt satisfied this was good enough. I planned to see her for a follow-up the next day, and I sent her home.

The next morning I came back to work. Just before lunchtime, I was sitting in the tiny office that I shared with two other registrars and a case manager. The phone on my desk rang. It was a call from another large university hospital.

"Is this Dr. Bonhoeffer?"

"Yes, speaking."

"This is Dr. Smith from Guy's Hospital. Do you remember..."

As soon as I heard those three words, they reverberated through my body like an electric shock. I knew very well that when another doctor is calling me from another hospital asking me if I remember something about a patient I have seen recently, it is not heralding good news. It means they either desperately need some information that I might have, or it means that I have made a mistake and they want to give me feedback. The tone in this doctor's voice sounded very much like it was the latter.

"... a young Afro-Caribbean girl who you saw yesterday? She was admitted this morning unconscious to our intensive care unit. We had to intubate and ventilate because of respiratory failure. We have taken X-rays, and we have found a handball-size tumor in her chest, which we believe to be non-Hodgkin lymphoma, based on rapid section histology."

This doctor was just calling as a courtesy to let me know that this girl, the girl I had misdiagnosed as having an acute asthma attack with no risk factors, this same girl for whom I had neglected to order an X-ray, this same girl who actually is at risk for this disease because of her age and ethnicity, actually had non-Hodgkin lymphoma. He was also aiming to gather some additional information I might have.

It was immediately obvious that I had made a terrible mistake. I felt ashamed. I had failed this innocent little girl in my professional capacity, and put her life at risk. The rush of adrenaline caused me to stand up involuntarily from my chair. My mind started to rush fast with ideas. How could I justify my decision? How can I make this okay? What could I do to find a solution for the situation?

There was no way out. She was now under someone else's care, where she was now being diagnosed and treated correctly.

For the rest of the day, I was devastated. I still had to do my rounds. I felt completely folded in on myself, cut off from everyone. I felt intimidated, shy, and nervous in my decision-making. I wasn't really present with the other children, with this story running around my head. The whole day I was exhausted, I didn't feel like doing anything. I was longing for a way to hide, to retreat and to reflect and to recover, but that was not possible. The next phone call came, the next nurse knocking on the door, the next patient to be seen. The high-pressure environment continued.

The hospital was in South London, and I was living in Walthamstow, in the north of London. This was actually a good idea, because it allowed for a long tube ride at the beginning and the end of every day: protected reading and reflection time. It was on the way home that I started to be able to think. Medically, what could I have done differently? What should I have done differently? Where had I failed? Could I have really known this? Should I have done the tests, no matter how it seemed? The deeper I went into this reflection, the more deeply I realized that it was my ignorance and sloppiness that had caused the situation, and nothing else. There was no excuse, and there was no defense, no one and nothing to blame.

I started to have pictures of this little girl in my mind. I saw her being intubated, I visualized her in the intensive care, I visualized her sister, and I imagined her parents. I could picture her shock, and her difficulty in breathing. Then I imagined how it would come out, sooner or later, that she had seen me. I could visualize everyone at the other hospital pointing at me saying, "It was him. He made the mistake."

I experienced a very contracted feeling of pressure in my chest that I would label as "guilt." I wanted just to curl up, like an embryo, and disappear. There was a burning sensation in my solar plexus. I felt so ashamed.

When I came home, I couldn't fall asleep easily. I kept seeing all the same pictures. I felt so small, and guilty. I was tossing about in the bed. "How can I deserve to sleep peacefully in my bed when this poor little girl is suffering because of me?" I wanted to get out of the bed, and rush to the hospital where she now was, and apologize to her and her family. My mind was going wild for hours, as I was tossing about from one side to the other, unable to fall deeply asleep.

Finally I did fall into a kind of sleep, and I had a dream. I was floating above the bed, and above the room, and I see myself tossing and turning in the bed below. I saw this young Swiss doctor, beating himself up so badly. I saw a young man desperately wanting to have a positive impact on others. I saw a young doctor who could not accept making mistakes. He deserved a break. And then, from this vantage point of the ceiling, I could see that this young doctor was deeply well-intentioned, he had simply made this one mistake.

In the morning, once I got out of bed, the feeling had changed. It was still a serious mistake, but now I could also forgive myself. I was very clear. I took a paper and a pen, and wrote some commitments. I resolved to do better in the future. I resolved to pay more attention to all the pieces of the puzzle, even if they don't freely fit my own ideas of what is going on. I made a resolve never again to shortcut on the tests but to explore all possible explanations. Throughout my career as a pediatrician, I have kept the promises that I wrote that day.

Although this was a painful experience for everybody, it was a very powerful learning experience for me. Almost fifteen years later, I had the chance to look at this again as Arjuna encouraged me to take this to the next level, extend the definition of "mistake," and learn from my everyday small mistakes in a proactive, conscious, loving, and very structured way. Here is Arjuna:

*

Hey, Hannah. Everybody makes mistakes sometimes, not just in medicine but in every field. If you make a mistake that affects someone else negatively (as happened here) or even that affects your own health negatively, it's absolutely natural to temporarily feel shame, regret, remorse, or to feel like a failure.

These feelings are very unpopular in our culture for several reasons. First, they used to be shoved down our throats until a few decades ago by religions, which thrived on people feeling permanently ashamed and guilty. So there was a backlash in the "new age" movement of the 1970s and '80s to heal ourselves from ever having these feelings. But you can easily throw the baby out with the bath water. If you feel ashamed and guilty all the time, obviously that would be toxic, and to be avoided. On the other hand, if you make a mistake that you'd rather not repeat, it is important to experience these feelings viscerally in the body, at least for a few minutes. If you think about a mistake only cognitively, the learning does not really land anywhere. We have to fully allow and experience that sinking, collapsing feeling in the chest, that feeling of, "Oh no, I can't believe I did that," in order for it to really turn into a valuable learning.

I recommend to myself, and to everyone I work with, to deliberately take a few minutes to reflect on mistakes at the end of every day. Five or ten minutes is enough to do the trick.

Here is the practice.

Toward the end of the day, whenever you officially finish work, take a few minutes for self-reflection. The ideal time is when the sun goes down, because it is the right kind of atmosphere, but this depends upon your work schedule.

Let yourself reflect upon the different things that happened during the day. This is not (only) about critical incidents. This is about anything you know you could have done better: in a way you now feel some twinge of regret.

There are many variations this could take:

~ It could be a time when you were abrupt with someone else, harsh or impatient.
~ It could be a time when you were careless with someone else's well-being.
~ It could be a time when lack of knowledge — or getting caught up in your concepts rather than looking with fresh eyes — put patients at risk, as in the story Jan describes.
~ It could also be a time when you were abrupt or careless with yourself and you didn't pay enough attention to the needs of your body.
Let yourself evoke this memory strongly enough that you feel it viscerally. This means that you don't just think about it, but you let it become a sinking, heavy feeling in your chest: the kind of feeling that we often

label as "shame" or "guilt" or "remorse." Stay in this feeling for just a few minutes.

Then you can deliberately recreate what happened to Jan spontaneously. You can zoom out a little bit, and observe yourself feeling guilty. You can remember your good intentions. You can remember that you are a good person, that you absolutely want to have the best effect on the greatest number of people. You can deliberately cultivate and practice feelings of self-forgiveness.

Finally, you can turn this into a learning. What would you do differently the next time? Given the opportunity to go through the same set of circumstances again, how would you make different choices?

Chapter Fifteen
Choose Your Role Models

Dear Hannah,

As you enter into residency, you will meet a whole variety of more senior colleagues, with much greater knowledge and experience than you. Nothing need prevent you from learning all you can from them. You will be able to shadow them, to work alongside them, and to observe not only what they know, but also how they interact with their patients. I want to talk to you here about how you can develop the best relationships with these potential role models and mentors.

You are being trained in an environment that is primarily driven by science. Empirical knowledge and objectivity are considered to be the highest values. Consequently, some of your teachers may not be as familiar with other components of healing that are more human and heart-based. Many of your teachers, who are much older than you, may have been trained with the idea that the medical professional is much more knowledgeable than the patient, which allows them to assert superiority and authority.

In this conventional system, medicine is purely objective. An injection of 10 mg of adrenalin will have the same effect, no matter who prescribes it, or who is operating the syringe. A blood pressure of 110/60 means the same, whoever took the measurement. Consequently, medicine has been reduced to a collection of objective statistics, measurements, and prescriptions. The practice of medical science has followed a very reductionist model, which establishes a definition of "normal," a set of deviations, which we call "illness," and then a series of standardized prescriptions for recovery.

We can find many medical cultures where the healthcare professional is not only a scientist but also a consultant on well-being in a much broader sense. In central Europe, doctors used to be monks. In other societies, like in Africa and Asia and South America, healers used to be shamans in their respective cultures, and they combined qualities of diagnosis and prescription as well as the more intuitive sense of a holistic well-being. This is why medicine was considered to be an art as well as a science, before this very questionable division occurred between art and science in academia.

What I am talking with you about in these letters — showing up fully and being present with your heart open, and connecting deeply with people as a vehicle of love — does not even show up on the radar in conventional medicine. It would not be true to say that most conventional doctors do not want this kind of connection; they have simply forgotten that it even exists. Very often, people did not get this kind of connection themselves. Even the highest authorities in the hospital may not have received the kind of loving attention, care, and real healing that I want to point you toward. So you have to forgive people. It would not be true to say that the people who are supervising you and teaching you know all about the wisdom of the heart, and then choose to reject it. It is simply the case that the heart atrophies when it has not been cared for properly, and when we have no example of how people can deeply care for each other. When all that people know — and all that they have been trained in — is a sterile, objective system which treats each patient as a number, it becomes almost impossible to imagine anything else.

Everyone you meet in the hospital is somehow doing their best, as they struggle through their lives. The people you meet professionally may not be having the greatest sex life, the greatest nourishment, the greatest food, they may not be feeling loved and appreciated at home. You cannot blame people. We have to understand that people do the best they can. It is simply important, as you enter the system, to listen to the calling of your heart and to realize that what you are being taught, and the system you are moving into, is very incomplete.

Hannah, you are under no obligation to be trained by more senior people, and then to copy what they tell you. You can do much better than the current system of medicine. You can change the system. You can transform the medical world simply by gently refusing to compromise your heart, and insisting upon a new standard of presence and care. You have to bring something from your side to make the situation complete, because there is a whole big piece missing that many of your teachers will not even know exists.

As you meet different senior doctors and teachers, it is important to have some standards to filter how much you want to be influenced. One is to recognize how knowledgeable someone is, and how useful it may be to absorb this knowledge for your own practice as a doctor. But you can also filter how healthy this person is. Do they exhibit a way of being in the world that you want to emulate? You need to be able to discriminate about who you can learn from, and who you need to have compassion for. Sometimes it will be exactly the same people.

Now let me tell you about two of my teachers, who influenced me in quite different ways.

*

When I was a resident, I was assigned to a hospital in Zürich. There was a very gifted surgeon there, a very senior man, who was in charge of the department of surgery.

At that time, someone in a position like this was almost always a highly decorated military officer. It was almost an inflexible requirement for anyone in a position of leadership, anywhere, to also have accumulated seniority in the military. From the age of eighteen to sixty-four, every man was required to serve in the military for two or three weeks every year. It was deemed that if you are a military officer who has accumulated seniority, you have strong leadership capabilities. Hard to believe today, but this is how it was.

So the head of the surgical department at the hospital was a highly decorated military man, and this was how he ran the operation. Every morning at 7:30 a.m. sharp, all the hospital staff lined up for inspection. You could see the clock going: 7:29 and 56 seconds... 57... 58... 59... "Good morning, everybody."

Then the day would begin. The entire surgical team would go into the theater and start operating on patients. Before lunchtime they would go and do their rounds. During lunch, they would find something to eat, if they were lucky; otherwise they would go to see more patients. In the afternoon they would go back to the theater. One team would stay on to operate and to deal with emergencies, and the other team would go back to the wards and do more rounds. The entire staff was living off the vending machine: cheap coffee, Snickers bars, Mars bars, and sandwiches. Many of them were smoking cigarettes.

The head of the department was either performing operations, or he went straight home. He never came to any team events or connected with us in any kind of personal way. He was always secluded in his private office. Nothing in his life seemed to be relational. Everyone in the hospital was a functional cog in his machine.

It was wintertime when I worked in this department. I had a flat in Zürich not too far from the clinic. I did not have to attend lectures anymore, so I wanted to make the best use of my time. I would drive to work in the car, and every night I would return. Typically I would leave the house at 6 o'clock in the morning, and I would come back around 11 o'clock or midnight. Several nights a week and two weekends out of the month, I was also on night shift, in addition to the work of the day. Sometimes, I would start work on Monday morning, and then work through until Thursday evening without a break. Then I would go home, sleep for six hours, and come back and continue. For the weekend, I would regularly stay at the hospital from Friday morning until Monday evening, without any break.

Obviously, there were times when I was so tired that I would just sit in a chair and immediately fall asleep. Often I did not go home, because just to take the effort to drive, open my blankets, and take off my clothes, and then have to come back the next morning, was completely overwhelming. There was always some corner where I could crash at the hospital for a twenty-minute nap.

I was the one holding the wound open in the operating theater, assisting the surgeons to do their jobs.

Sometimes I would lose tension, as I almost fell asleep standing at the operating table without moving for hours. Then the head of the surgical department would take the steel scissors and whip my hand hard.

Please understand, this man was a medical genius. Whenever he said something medical or educational, it was pure gold. He was a phenomenal surgeon and much respected and admired by his patients. I learned so much from him.

But, as a human being, he was very difficult for me. In the many months that I worked there, he never said one word of appreciation. Not one time. He was quick with extremely harsh criticism. If he asked me to do something, and I did not immediately understand, or know how to do it, he would send me away from the operating table. "Now, you leave the table. I will have to do this alone. Go and read about it in a book. When you are properly educated, you can come back. The next time, you'd better be prepared." He used to make a big display out of these situations, so the experience had maximum humiliation value. I was one of many experiencing this. When it was my turn, other members of the team would watch, and later say, "You poor guy. This time you got it." For sure, I spent the rest of the nights reading and preparing the theater list for the next day.

Once I caught a cold. I had a high fever, of close to 40°C., 104°F. I had a splitting headache, a blocked nose; I could hardly drink, my throat was so sore. I came to him and said, "I think it may be best for me to take a day off to recover." I was also concerned for my effect on the patients. His response was always the same in these situations. "There are only two reasons why a surgeon does not come into work. Either you are being operated on yourself, or you are dead. If neither of these qualifications is met, I expect you in theater." One of the top physicians was also a great skier. He had a skiing accident, and fractured his leg below the knee. He had to be operated on, to have it screwed back together. Then he was in a cast. But he was also not allowed to take time off work. "What is your problem?" the head surgeon asked. "You can just lean on the cast while you operate. It's very convenient; you will not even need to use a chair. Just lean on your cast, and do your job."

I had to work these crazy long hours, under these crazy conditions, being criticized every day. Several times I broke down crying in theater with tears rolling into my mask. The chief surgeon did not appear to notice. I was dizzy, I was seeing strange colors and hallucinations. But he continued his criticism, always requiring more.

It was at the end of this phase of my life that I decided to go to India. Working at the Sassoon General Hospital, I met Mme. Phadke. She was also one of my most influential teachers, but in a vastly different way.

Madam Phadke was about fifty years old, a very tall, beautiful Indian lady, always adorned in flowing colorful saris. Wherever she appeared people would turn their heads, not because of her beauty, but because of her incredible presence. When I met her the first time, I was waiting for her in the corridor. She walked toward me, to welcome me to the hospital, followed by a trail of junior and senior physicians. Whenever they had time, everybody in the hospital would shadow her, and learn from her. Everybody admired her for her incredible wealth of knowledge that nobody could even come close to.

But we were also mesmerized by the way she was making diagnoses, and relating to patients. It allowed her to be very connected, but also very fast and efficient. Her colleagues would discuss this endlessly: how does she figure it out? How does she know? Did she nail it again? When everybody else was perplexed about a complex case, and how to resolve it, she would come into the room and within a few minutes would have the solution.

Often, this happened through being with the patient without saying or doing much. It was almost as if she was sensing the patient, as if she herself was the diagnostic tool.

After this period of "feeling" the patient, she would simply ask a few direct and pointed questions.

"So my impression is…," she would say, "this is what is going on with you." Every single time the patient would respond "Yes!" There was an immediate acknowledgment and confirmation. This came from a visceral level in the patient. The patient has no way to confirm a medical diagnosis, particularly a complex one. Usually, with other doctors, there was confusion, and questions, and worries. But whenever she explained her diagnosis to the patient, it was met with full acceptance and immediate understanding, as if they could feel this is true.

I shadowed her a lot, so I saw this very often. Even the senior physicians would come to her, saying, "Look, we have this real issue, we need your help." Then they would relax just from being in her presence: the conversation would change in quality. There was more listening, more of a shared calm finding of solutions, rather than an excited solving of problems. It was the same for patients: people in pain, in agony, fear, and worries. When she showed up they could immediately feel that, "This is someone who is here for me. I am being seen, and I am being taken care of. I am being heard, and I am being taken seriously." This, combined with her medical authority, was what put people at ease.

She treated me and all the other doctors with great respect. The day when it was time for me to leave, she summoned me to the Dean's office, to meet with her and four of her top people in the department. "Oh my God," I was thinking. "What did I do wrong?"

"So tell me what you have learned," she asked. I told her about some of the things I had experienced during my time in India. One was that the kids I saw dying every day were dying of waterborne diseases, lack of hygienic conditions, and lack of running water. They were dying of vaccine-preventable diseases, like measles.

"You are a young doctor from Switzerland," she said. "I am regularly in and out of Geneva with the World Health Organization. With what you have seen here, I ask you to go back to Switzerland, and go to the World Health Organization, let them know what you have seen and address these issues. Let's make sure that we make progress in these areas. As you can see, this is not just something on paper, but something very real that affects real people."

Madam Phadke was my inspiration for twenty years working in vaccine safety and with the World Health Organization, and she is a role model for Heart-Based Medicine.

*

As you go through your medical career, it will be very helpful and important for you to establish healthy role models. There are three criteria that I have found very useful in determining whom to turn to as a role model, and why.

First, there are role models who will be influential for you because of what they know and their skills. This would include the head of the surgical department I just described. Sometimes, you will meet people who know so much that you can kindly forgive and overlook their personality.

Second, there will be role models who influence you because of their impressive level of health, in a multidimensional way. You will meet people who are physically, emotionally, and mentally healthy (they have the capacity to think clearly in an out-of-the-box way), as well as spiritually healthy. These kinds of role models may or may not have the level of knowledge that we described above. But they become examples of the kind of human being that you want to grow into.

Third, there are role models who demonstrate how to create extraordinary levels of rapport and connection with patients. These are the healthcare professionals who engender trust, connection, and relaxation in the patients. In an earlier letter, I described to you my friend Roger who adopted one of his patients. He had this capacity to immediately set patients at ease.

Occasionally, you may meet the rare and inspiring human being who demonstrates all three of these qualities at the same time. When you do, enjoy and absorb their every movement and gesture. You will not be sleep deprived, I promise.

Arjuna has shared a great deal with me about the art of building wonderful relationships with role models. He even wrote an entire chapter about this in one of his books, which you can read here: heartbasedmedicine.org/registerbook. Here he is:

*

Hey, Hannah. When you meet a doctor or any kind of medical professional who strikes you as an inspiring example of any of the three criteria above, I suggest that you do one simple thing. People are very busy. A lot of people feel that they are very important. But everyone has one little weak spot. When we were all growing up, at one time or another we were delivered this maxim: "There is no such thing as a free lunch." Everyone has been indoctrinated in one way or another to believe that a free lunch is a miracle. Consequently, however busy someone is, if you offer to buy them lunch, it is very difficult to refuse.

When you find someone in your medical training who you feel really impressed by, you simply need to deliver this message, either verbally, or as an email or a written note. "You have been an incredible inspiration to me. I have a few questions I would love to ask you. May I invite you out to lunch?" Hannah, I have made this little overture to some very busy and celebrated people. I have never been turned down yet. Of course, make sure that you take your role model out to a really nice place. McDonald's or Taco Bell would not be good considerations.

Once you sit down together, it is a good idea to ask your role model if they would mind you placing a little voice recorder on the table. This may be an opportunity that does not come again, and you want to be able to savor it afterwards. Here are a few good questions to ask someone who is an inspiration to you:

"How did you get started? What was your moment of initial motivation?"

"What is your greatest passion today? What is new and exciting for you?"

"What are the biggest mistakes you have made? What would you not to do again?"

"I have this idea/project/vision I have been working on. I'd really like to get your feedback and your opinion."

"Who were the greatest role models for you? In order to be a really great doctor, who would you most recommend me to meet or study?"

"What is the most important advice you would give to someone like me, just starting out to be a doctor?"

Developing relationships like this with the very best doctors you can find on the planet will be an enormous boost for you to shift your identity toward becoming this kind of great healer yourself.

Chapter Sixteen
Connect With the Infinite

Dear Hannah,

I have kept the best for last. In this letter, I want to talk to you about the thing (or perhaps the no-thing) that has absolutely made the most difference to me. In previous letters, I talked about some of the things that are unlikely to be covered in your medical training. But I doubt that you will ever hear a whisper about what I want to talk to you about today... even though it has been a massive part of human experience and development, and has been influential on every culture, in every tradition, in every period of history. It may be surprising when we get into this topic together, but as I said: it has made such a huge difference to me that I could not leave it out of my letters to you.

Connect With the Infinite

This is the secret sauce.

Most of my letters to you have contrasted what you learn in medical school with the disposition that you bring to your patients. This includes the way you take care of yourself, the way that you listen, and the way that you question your habitual thinking. But this letter goes much deeper, Hannah. This is about who you really are.

It is a topic that is very difficult to write about. It really needs to be experienced. It is like introducing the topic of color in a black-and-white movie or trying to introduce the idea of waking up within a dream.

*

Now I want to tell you another story during my time in India after I had been working in the surgical team I told you about in the previous chapter.

I was so exhausted, I hardly knew my name. I knew that I would have to either pull out of medical school, or completely change my environment. I wanted to go somewhere where I didn't know anyone, and no one knew me, where the culture and everything was as different as possible. India operates at a different pace: there was time to rest and reset, there was time to sleep. There was time for contemplation and meditation.

I got a position as an intern in the pediatric department at the Sassoon General Hospital, in Pune. I had a friend who was already living in that area, who was involved with the Rajneesh ashram. He told me that when I arrived I could stay with him for a few days, in Koregaon Park, and get settled.

From the very beginning, I used to get up at 4 o'clock in the morning, and just sit in the park quietly. There was a beautiful statue of Krishna, in the middle of a lush garden. I would just find a spot to sit on the ground in the early morning. Then I would go get myself a masala chai and half a papaya with lime for breakfast. There was an Ayurvedic clinic nearby, where the doctor was very gifted with panchakarma treatment, massages, and herbal medicine. The doctor there was a great teacher for me, a role model of living a healthy life as a healer.

After a few weeks, my friends introduced me to Kiran, an older Indian man, who was holding meetings for a handful of people in his house. He helped me to see beyond my desperate and locked-in separate sense of self with great patience and love, and to relax some of the suffering I had experienced in medical school during the months before in Switzerland. He supported me to remember my initial motivation for becoming a doctor, and caring for people. He recommended that I enter more deeply into a practice of meditation every day. He suggested, "Why don't you get up early in the morning, when everything is still quiet, and the day starts, and just sit and be quiet." And that is what I did.

Day by day, I could feel the tension was dropping away, and all my ideas about who I am, and where I need to go, and what I need to do, and what I am good at, and what I am feeling, were dissolving. I was discovering a more relaxed and loving approach to myself and my environment.

My room looked out onto the Mula-Mutha River. On the other side of the river, I could see the water buffaloes were grazing in the morning as the mist was rising. It was India at its most beautiful. I could smell the fires of the burning ghats, where they burn bodies of people who have died. Across the river, I could see the Aga Khan Palace, where Gandhi had been held in prison.

My room was very simple. There was nothing but a mattress on the marble floor, a Nelson textbook of pediatrics, a standard Ayurvedic textbook, and a simple shelf for my clothes. I wore the same clothes all the time, even at the hospital: simple thin white cotton pants, with a drawstring, and a white shirt that extended almost to the knee. The walls of the room had been painted with a chalk-based whitewashed paint that would rub off easily on your hands when you touched it. Although the building was relatively new, it already looked old, as was very common in India. It had very dark brown Colonial-style doors. The room had a door that opened toward the river, but there was no balcony. Outside the door was simply a metal railing. So in the mornings, I would open the door, and then sit in meditation on the floor.

One morning, I was sitting on my cushion, with my shawl around me, simply looking over the river into the moorlands. There was a thick mist close to the ground, and the water buffaloes were moving in slow motion, grazing as the day was breaking. There was a very special light, which you only see in India. It created an extraordinarily beautiful scene; everything was still and serene, yet deeply alive. It was very quiet.

It was a day just like every other day. I was sitting, meditating, feeling more and more relaxed. Then something completely let go, and there was no more control. My eyes were still seeing the landscape, but there was no person there. There was no difference between what was being seen, and the one seeing. The sense of me was gone. There was no localized observer experiencing anything, there was just a pervading oneness. There was no separation between who I am, and what my senses were collecting, or what was reflecting upon that.

I could still see the landscape, I could still smell the scent from the burning ghats, I could still hear the occasional sound of a motor rickshaw. I wasn't exactly deliberately "looking," it was more like a completely relaxed gazing without intention.

There was a sense of integration, of oneness, and actually being an expression of this same life energy: the same life force that is the dawn, that is the meadows, that is the fire consuming bodies at the burning ghat, that is the water buffaloes grazing, that is the cockroaches. I was a part of this expression of life, rather than looking at it as a separate observer. My body did not end with the skin. It did not have a clear starting and stopping point or delineation.

This ended with a sudden jolt.

"Whoa! What just happened?" I asked myself. "I just completely lost the sense of self I am used to."

There was nobody there, and then suddenly there was the sense of someone there again. A seemingly eternal moment of peace was followed by a moment of fear, effervescing up within the peace.

A few hours later I called Kiran, and asked him what was going on. He was very sweet; he simply said, "Great. Just return back to your meditation cushion."

This moment changed my life in many ways. Immediately, in the days following, it changed the way I saw patients and health and healing. It changed the way I touched people, and it changed the way that I experienced death.

I saw children die every day in the Sassoon hospital. This experience changed the way that I related to these families, to the mothers and to the children. I also found a different relationship to the burning ghats. I started to experience death and life as part of the same expression. I met many mothers in the hospital who had just lost their child, or who were about to lose their children, but they also had an attitude toward death that was different from what I had been used to in Europe.

That moment has opened the possibility of being together with someone at an extreme moment of life. When a mother is losing an infant, it is a very intense, very alive, a no-pretense situation. I can look at this from the outside, as an educated medical professional, and share with them what I have learned in medical school, but what became possible after this moment was that the gate was open to really connect and to share the experience as one. The sense of a doctor and a mother as separate was only one level. Just underneath it there was no separation. There was oneness.

Previous to this moment, there was a young doctor named Jan, there was a mother, there was a child, as three separate entities. They could communicate with each other, across the gap. Looked at in this way, after the death of a child, that small entity was gone... forever. I could try to build bridges between Jan as a separate entity and the grieving mother as another entity. After this moment, the feeling of being separate was much less. Somewhere, deep down, I knew that it is fundamentally a lie. Relating to the mother holding her dead child, or seeing the child lying next to her in a baby cot, there was less of a feeling of being separate, and more of a feeling of being one. There was less of a feeling of one person relating to another, and more of a feeling of the relating happening within the same space. It was a feeling of being together without boundaries.

*

In an earlier letter, I talked to you about the importance of feeding both wolves: the knowledge-hungry, empirical-science-and-data-driven wolf that gets fed in the University Hospital, and the second wolf, which is hungry for presence and connection. There is no better way to feed the second wolf than this. It's like superfood. Everything else is helpful, but this is the specialty of the chef.

This experience happened quite spontaneously. I did not intend for it to occur exactly in this way. Years later when much of this had become buried under the clutter of a busy life, I recommended for Jessica to attend a weekend event with Arjuna, before we started the coaching together. They did a practice that weekend called "Radical Awakening." When Jessica came home, she had experienced exactly the same thing that happened for me in India.

Arjuna has made this question central to his work, and the way he has trained coaches, for almost the last thirty years. He has engaged tens of thousands of people in this kind of inquiry, and the answers they give follow almost exactly the same pathways every time.

Connect With the Infinite

Let me hand this over to Arjuna, and he will tell you how he has been able to guide people to experience the same thing that happened to me, both one on one and in groups.

*

Hey, Hannah, it is true. Just the briefest moment of this kind of "awakening" changes everything. I had a moment like this myself about thirty years ago, and it became the very foundation of all the work that I have done with people since. Just as Jan mentioned, this happened for him spontaneously and naturally, but it can also be easily facilitated. Let's explore it together now.

In this moment, you are holding a book or an e-reader in your hand. You can see squiggly hieroglyphics on a white page. Is that true? If you look up for a moment, I am sure you can see other things as well: shapes, colors, textures, and movement. If I look up from the desk in my house I can see trees, and the sunlight moving through the trees. What can you see from where you are?

Now I am going to ask you a series of questions. As you hear or read each question, please pause for a moment, long enough to find out what is the honest and accurate answer for you.

The first question: **do you need to think** in order to see an object that is in front of you? For example, hold up your hand in front of your face. Look at the hand. Now that the hand is here, to see the hand, just to see it, not to understand or compare or give it meaning, does it require any thinking on your part?

Now look at something else. Look at this star here, for example:

☆

Unlike words, the star has no meaning. It is just a shape. To see it, just to see it, **is thinking required**? Or is it possible to fully see the shape before you without the need for thought?

Is it possible that seeing in fact occurs without thinking?

*

In the same way, **does it require any effort, or decision**, to see an object or a shape once it is already in front of you? Take a look at the star again:

☆

Once you have turned the attention to it, does it then require any effort or decision to see what is already here? Take a moment to look around, wherever you are. See the colors. See the movement. See the shapes. Does it require any effort or decision to see what is already in front of you?

Is it possible that seeing also occurs free of decision or effort?

And finally, **is there any time delay**, in your subjective experience, between the object being there and your experience of the object? You need to rely here on your own subjective experience, not what you think or have learned conceptually. When you see the star:

☆

... do you notice any time delay between the star being here and the experience of the star being here? Is it possible that seeing also happens outside of time?

Noticing this about seeing, which is happening now, and now, and now, consider whether it is possible that seeing is actually happening all the time, free of thinking, free of effort, free of decision, free of time.

Could you relax, even now, into being that which is seeing shapes and colors and movement?

Could you relax into being that now?

What is *that*, which we loosely refer to as "me," which is seeing in this moment? Who, or what, is experiencing this moment?

What Can You Hear?

In the same way, let's investigate together the nature of hearing. Listen for a moment to the sounds you can hear around you.

When you hear a sound, like a passing car, or a bird outside the window, **do you have to think to hear the sound**? Or would it be true to say that hearing is free of thinking?

As you hear a sound, any sound, **do you have to make an effort** to hear the sound that is already here? Do you say to your body, "OK, start to hear sounds?" Or might it be true that hearing is also effortless, decision-less?

Do you notice any time delay, in your own subjective experience, between the sound and the experience of the sound?

Take a moment to really investigate this for yourself. Hear the sounds now. And notice the process of hearing itself. Does hearing require thought, decision, effort, or time?

Could you relax now into being that which is hearing?

Who is it, or what is it, that is actually experiencing this very moment?

Feel the Sensations in the Body

Finally, we can ask the same questions about the sensations that are happening right now in your body. Take a moment to scan your body. Perhaps you can notice the moisture inside your mouth. Perhaps you can feel sensations of tension or relaxation.

In just the same way, when a sensation is present, **does it require any thought to notice the sensation? Does it require any effort or decision** to be aware of a sensation in the body, once the sensation is already there? **Is there any time delay**, in your subjective experience, between the sensation and the experience of the sensation?

Does feeling require any thought, effort, decision, or time? Or is feeling also just happening on its own?

Could you relax into being that which is seeing, hearing, and feeling in this very moment, now?

Who is it, or what is it, that is noticing shapes, sounds, and physical sensations in this moment?

Who, or what, is experiencing this moment?

If you took a tape measure, how big is it?

Although it hears sounds, does it in itself hear any sound?

Was it ever born?

Could it die?

Is it male or female?

Is it German or Swiss or American?

Now, could you relax even more deeply into just being this, which hears and sees and feels?

Could you allow yourself to become even more curious about the nature of this which you are, when you put aside — just for a moment — the personal story of "me" moving through time?

Take some time to investigate this before we continue.

Connect With the Infinite

You might like to pause now and go watch the video I have made for you, or listen to the audio recording, both of which guide you into this inquiry. This may deepen your experience.

*

Since 1991, I have asked this same series of questions to tens of thousands of people, not as an intellectual exercise, but as a genuine inquiry to find out what is true, from direct experience. Hopefully, you have had a chance now to find out what is true for you. Let's compare notes on what you discovered for yourself, even if it was only the tiniest taste, and what tens of thousands of other people have discovered as well.

People describe what they discover when they go look for that which is experiencing this moment in various ways. Consciousness... Spaciousness... Presence... Awareness...

Like a signpost that has the word "Rome" written on it, these words are pointing to something much bigger than words or concepts. The sign is not the city. These words are pointing toward a mysterious vastness, empty of content, but full of love and presence. It is this vast presence that is actually experiencing this moment.

For sure, there is also a story here, of a person born in time, and who will also die in time. Both of these exist simultaneously. The important difference is that the story requires thought, whereas the recognition of the presence is free of thought.

Sometimes people say, "I am experiencing this moment. I am. It is me." It is now necessary to investigate this "I" itself. What is it? Does it have any size? Does it have any color? Does it make any sound? Can it be found, from direct experience? Generally, when we investigate in this way, we discover that we have been using the words "I," "me," "mine," and "myself " for our whole lives without really knowing exactly what these words are referring to. When we investigate the "I," when we go look for it, it cannot be found, it is only a thought, or a concept, and then the inquiry leads us directly to the spaciousness of consciousness itself.

When people have a glimpse of their "true nature" in this way, — as vast, spacious, silent, and completely present — the question often comes up, "How can I keep this in my day-to-day life?" A good coach will help you to discover that this is not the most useful question to ask. A better question would be, "Is it actually possible to make this spaciousness go away in my day-to-day life?" Try it now. Move your hand from left to right. That is a movement, just like all the other movements that you make every day in your life. Did the movement make any difference to the awareness of the movement, to the spaciousness itself?

Go ahead and think any thought you choose. It could be a "positive" thought or a "negative" thought. It doesn't matter. Think any thought you like. Does the thought cause that which is aware of thought to disappear? Does it actually make any difference to the presence itself? Whatever thought arises, there can also be awareness of that thought, and that awareness does not change. That is who you are.

You can conjure up any kind of emotion. Experience the emotion, and then simply notice that you are also aware of the emotion. The emotion makes no difference to the presence.

It is a great practice to spend the rest of your life seeing if there is anything you can experience, think, or feel that could actually make any difference to this vast silent presence itself. You can try bungee jumping, skydiving, or running with the bulls. Wherever you are, there is also awareness of what is happening. The awareness does not change.

Of course, historically this kind of inquiry has been the domain of mysticism, and hence bleeds over into religion, and dogma and beliefs, which makes it an unlikely bedfellow for scientific inquiry. Hence, the inquiry into the purely subjective: the nature of consciousness itself, has been deemed irrelevant to science and also to medicine.

However, this is essentially important to everything you do as a doctor. In any moment that you have just a taste of the nature of consciousness itself, independent of things you see, and hear, and feel, and think about, something incredible happens. You feel a rush of energy, you are suddenly bathed in a refreshing wave of peace and sanity, you feel happy for no reason. You feel love for no reason. It is the deepest and most thorough reboot that could be possible.

Chapter Seventeen
Conclusion

Dear Hannah,

This will be my last of these letters to you, and it is going to be a short one.

It was not always easy for me to write these letters. Of course, although each and every word is written primarily for you, Hannah, as my goddaughter, I am aware that there are so many hundreds of thousands of other young doctors like you all over the world, and it has always been my intention in founding Heart-Based Medicine to support as many young, inspired doctors as possible.

A few years ago, a part of me was feeling quite comfortable and secure. I had a good position at the hospital, I had become a recognized expert in the field of vaccine safety, and I was regularly working with the Centers for Disease Control, the World Health Organization. I have a lovely family, and three healthy young children. Why rock the boat? Why stick my neck out?

In sharing the principles of Heart-Based Medicine with colleagues and other health care professionals, I have met with a variety of responses. Many people have cheered me on, wanting to collaborate, encouraging me that this is a message whose time has come. Others took it all with a more cynical, dry, and ironic sense of humor.

I happen to know you well, because you are Dominik's daughter. As your godfather, I feel deeply compelled to do anything and everything I can to support your well-being. But how many other young doctors are there, just like you, all over the world, each and every year, starting out their medical career filled with optimism and compassion? As a professor at the University, I meet such young doctors each and every day. Many of these young doctors become exhausted and cynical before the training is over. I realize that this is not so much because of anything that was misguided about their idealism, it is about a medical system that does not sufficiently culture the natural human aspiration to care with compassion: to allow ourselves to love.

In the last letter I sent to you, I shared with you a moment in India where the clouds parted, and I had a glimpse of "true nature," deeper than the usual procession of conditioned thoughts and reactive feelings.

Whenever anyone arrives at the taste of recognizing who they really are, outside of the activity of thinking and emotion, they use very similar language. People will sometimes say that what remains is simply "consciousness," or "awareness," or "infinity," but they also frequently use another word. People also say that what remains, deeper than thinking and emotion, is love. It means that who you really are, beyond the story of a localized me, is love itself.

We all of us frequently use the word "love." We say "I love you." All the time. It means something when we say it. We all have a subjective experience, which we call "love." And yet, although it is one of the most central human experiences, it has never been scientifically measured. No one has yet developed an accurate gauge to determine if love is really present or not. But I know when I feel love. You know when you feel love. Everybody knows it.

If I ask you, "Do you love your father?" I know that you would say yes. And then, if I produced some data and told you, "This is the cutting-edge love-meter and it says that you don't love your father at all, and that you never have," you would probably, like most people, conclude that the machine is not adequate to measure love. For almost everybody, empirical data would not cause them to doubt their experience of something as fundamental as love.

Love is at the essence of what gives life meaning and depth. As you can tell from the many letters I have written to you, it is love that I believe has the tremendous possibility to heal. But love in medicine has also suffered from the valid and legitimate increase in empirical data.

When we realize the healing potential of love, we are faced with a central confusion. On one hand, it can seem that love is something we are missing, and that we must add to ourselves. It is something to learn and cultivate. There is some truth to this: you can learn to behave in a more loving way, you can learn to express more love, you can learn to be with other people in a way that they feel more loved. On the other hand, we can recognize, in glimpses and snapshots, that love is who we are. It is fundamental. It is what remains when we relax the tension of not-love. In that way, love is not different from presence, or consciousness. These are just different words for a fundamental ground of being.

Hannah, I have known you since you were born. Almost from the very first day, I have seen you in so many situations in your life where you felt free, relaxed, comfortable, loved, and taken care of. As soon as you remember so many moments from your childhood when you felt completely at ease and loved and at peace, that is what I mean by "love is who you are." I am not talking about some spiritual achievement. It is something very simple, that you already know very well: these moments in your life when everything relaxes, when you don't need anything from anyone, whether there is simply joy without a cause, and you are present.

With all of life's busyness and pressures, with your studies and your work in the hospital, it becomes easy to skip over and to forget these moments. It is easy to forget the value of those moments when you relax as love. It is easy to get disconnected from the nourishing quality of those moments, the way that they reset us and reconnect us. As a doctor, I have learned that it is not just a luxury to feed such moments, but a necessity. It is the foundation of being a healer, and not just a technician. You rediscover these moments when you are deeply connected with yourself, with your friends, your family, and with your patients.

Whenever you meet a patient in that place of being love, you naturally see your patients for who they are. When you rest as love, you see love looking back at you. Then there is no difference essentially between you and the other. This is, of course, completely outside the curriculum of any medical school in the world. It will completely change the way you look at health and disease, and completely change the quality of what you are doing. You step out of the framework of separation: where you are the doctor with the knowledge, and the patients are the ones with the problem. You enter a common ground where you are both together on the journey to healing and wholeness and completion. Then you are both in a learning disposition, you are both students of this life.

In order to become a more viable healer, in order to become a more loving presence, in order to become someone who has a healing influence on your patients, it is not necessary to change yourself, or to improve yourself. I have discovered that it is more important to relax deeply into yourself, deeply enough that you know yourself, in your essence, to be love itself.

Conclusion

Perhaps this is the most important, as well as the most unconventional and scary, thing I could say to any young doctor. But to be complete and authentic with you, this must also be said.

These letters were something like a calling for me. I knew that if I could have an impact on you by writing them, as my goddaughter, and even just a few other young people like you, to stay more connected with the integrity of their own hearts, then there was no way to ignore the calling.

The future of medicine is much more in your hands than in mine. In fifteen or twenty years I will be preparing to retire from my professional career. You are just starting yours. You will come to your own conclusions and understanding, way beyond anything that I have discovered in my career. I hope that you will hear these letters as an encouragement not to listen to me, or to any other external authority, but to trust in, and foster, the wisdom and intuition that is to be found in the temple of your own heart.

With all my love,
Your godfather, Jan

Afterword

Dear Hannah:

When I met your godfather in San Francisco at the Heart-Based Medicine Conference, I quickly felt I had met my twin. We were both insisting that the practice of medicine should be fun and precious. We also agreed these values are not what we get in medical school. I think he wrote this book for you in the hope that medical school did not hurt you in your pursuit to become your ultimate fantasy doctor. What I like about this book is that not only does it show that he wants to protect you from the monster known as "modern medical practice," but he also wants to protect the sacred, poetical, playful practice of medicine. This will allow you to be the kind of doctor you dream about.

I have loved every second of my fifty-two years in medicine; I love people and I love to care. I want to be with suffering so that I can love and guide playfully. I do this so a patient and their family can have a delightful journey toward wellness… whatever the consequences. As doctors, we know we cannot erase the horrors and anxieties that float into people's lives. However, we will get to know patients and their families. With this knowledge, we will be able to ease suffering. We aren't able to dive into our patients' concerns in the time limits we are taught in medical school. Every person is complicated; the more we know, the more creative our solution! Remember: a person is not their disease. Also, our desire for closeness is not just for the patient; the more we know, the deeper our understanding of humanity. You have a carte blanche for giving hugs and for playfulness.

When your godfather is offering self-care advice, please do it as you know best. And ask friends if you want more help. And I want to add one more thing to his self-care advice. As the deep philosopher Mary Poppins once sang: "In every job that must be done, there is an element of fun. You find that fun and the job's a game." Finding this fun is as important as love, especially to prevent burnout. Have toys in your pocket, memorize songs and poetry, and use them all, indiscriminately. And don't forget improvisation! You can always say, "I'm sorry" or "Whoops!"

From the moment I decided to practice medicine, I decided that I wanted to be fun to be with and to be fun to die with. Because of my focus on love and fun, I never feel depressed or burned out. Instead of taking antidepressants, I clown with others and invite others to clown with me to remind all of us that we are connected. I'm a clown who became a doctor, and I'm offering the idea of clowning to you as well.

Please, take care of yourself. Be an example of care for others. Have great friendships, wild exercises, find sacred moments of calmness, and follow your interests and hobbies as far as you are able. Connection to others, a lush romance with nature, and being well fed with the arts are three cornerstones of mental health. As you dream, find friends, working in healthcare, who share your dream, and work together. We need beautiful models of change.

During your medical life, you will face the most drastically unhealthy world in our shared history. The earth, our most fragile patient, has been diagnosed with symptoms relating to a changing climate that needs intensive care. When it's difficult to find a single healthy country in a sea of greed, we need good medicine. Your example of positive change will go a long way.

Afterword

So, go to it, Hannah! Every so often, drop me a line to let me know how it's going. By listening and following your godfather's advice, you'll reach your fantasy. Whee!

In Peace,
Patch Adams, MD
Director, Gesundheit! Institute

For More Information:
heartbasedmedicine.org

Acknowledgements

So many have contributed to the journey that has led to this book that it seems impossible to name them all.

Both authors are deeply grateful for the patience and trust of our beloved partners to allow for the countless hours of diving deep into uncharted territory of health care.

We thank the many colleagues who shared their stories in the last three years of conversation about bringing more heart into medicine. Their often unspoken suffering and pain have encouraged us to climb higher in a quest to crystallize the opportunities to evolve together beyond the current paradigm.

We are grateful for the learnings from the children we care for. They continue to be our teachers and mentors to see the needs of the next generation of health care professionals and patients.

A preliminary manuscript of this book was titled *Dear Hannah* and shared at the Heart-Based Medicine Summit 2019 in San Francisco. Both authors are deeply grateful for the critical review and feedback on this preliminary edition by the conference participants.

There are no words for all the learning from the patients whose stories we share in this book – with names and places changed to protect their privacy. They have paved the way for our work in the translational research lab at Heart-Based Medicine where we investigate love as the expression of unified field healthcare.

Huge thanks to Flo Selfman of Words à la Mode for proofreading. The cover design was created by Heike Becker of heikebecker.design, who is a much valued and inspiring member of the Heart-Based Medicine Team, co-creating the vision and mission from the beginning.

We are grateful to our publicist Drew Gerber at Wasabi Publicity for his honorable and exemplary ways of holding up the professional standard during times of radical change in the publishing industry.

Acknowledgements

*

Jan says:

Some key mentors and guides are highlighted in the stories of my personal journey. Some of their names and places are changed to protect their privacy. Among the countless, let me highlight here: I am eternally indebted to my parents Rosmarie and Walter Bonhoeffer who, with their relentless, loving care, have prepared the ground for basic trust in life and the fundamentally good nature of people.

Kiran, a tilemaker living with his family and giving Satsang in his backyard in Mukund Nagar Pune, India, and all over the world, who so clearly guided the way to tapping into the unified field.

My first academic teacher and Neuroscientist Prof. J. Glees, in Göttingen, and Prof. Durrer, University of Basel, who enthusiastically kindled the awe of medical students for the creation we live in and taught us the principles of what is referred to as one-medicine and system health today.

Mme. Phadke, Dean of B. J. Medical College, Pune, India, sealed my journey in paediatrics as a most aspired-to role model of medical impeccability and radiant care for each of the hundreds of children under her care every day.

I also bow to my teachers at John Radcliffe Hospital, Oxford: Prof. Peter Sullivan, who opened my eyes to the well-being of children far beyond the science and the bedside care he exemplified, and Prof. Richard Moxon, who held up the torch of scientific rigor and professional distance while deeply caring for the health of each child. Prof. Ulrich Heininger held my hand as my mentor during residency and had my back as Head of Department as a young attending and researcher on his team. He exemplified the crucial art of compassionate listening and seeing the world through the family's eyes.

I am indebted to the hospital clowns, who constantly invited me to smile as they caught me live in action and stuck in inner contractions, stuck beliefs, and seriousness.

Indeed, also, my beloved wife Jessica belongs in this list as she is also a professional colleague – a Developmental Pediatrician who introduced me to seeing the world through the eyes of the children at a much deeper level.

My wife Jessica has also generously supported the countless hours and night shift calls with Arjuna and

Acknowledgements

colleagues in the East and West of the globe with her patience and readiness to sacrifice some of our time as a couple, parents, and partners in the Child Health Center Youkidoc Kindergesundheit in Basel. I feel blessed and supported in my calling beyond the family. And here are Enya, Nael, and Naima, our three dearly loved children, who are my daily inspiration and soul nourishment. Their hugs, kisses, and wisdom whispered into my ear before going to bed give me the strength and courage to help evolve the current medical paradigm. They repeatedly forgive me for being away far too often while serving their peers in clinics and want to know all about it. I am stunned by a kind of satisfaction they express for contributing to a deeper cause beyond their immediate needs while feeling the pains of relinquishing daddy time.

I am profoundly grateful to Dominik von Lukowicz, my childhood friend, for his trust in me as a godfather to his daughter. Hannah, you have been a burst of sunshine in my life, and the inspiration for this first book on Heart-Based Medicine. I have learned so much from your critical review, inspiring comments and our conversations in a series of evening calls on the letters.

This book was born out of my relationship with my coach, Arjuna Ardagh. Because he was holding a trusted space and encouraged me to follow my inner voice, I was able to focus on the core message of the book, as well as the many stories and learnings from thirty years of clinical experience. As a masterful wordsmith with twelve books to his name, he turned the recordings of our dialogues into a manuscript with his unique poetic flourish. This book was truly a co-creation and a synergy of complementary skill sets at every step of the way.

*

Arjuna says:

Generally I have been in the habit of writing a hefty list of acknowledgments at the end of my previous books. This time I will narrow it down to just one name.

Thank you, Jan, for being my co-creator, my very pliable and self-reflective coaching client, my true friend and brother, and my inspiration for a better world.